# DIGESTIVE INTELLIGENCE

## INTELLIGENCE

A HOLISTIC VISION OF YOUR SECOND BRAIN

D0029456

# DIGESTIVE
# INTELLIGENCE

## A HOLISTIC VISION OF YOUR SECOND BRAIN

IRINA MATVEIKOVA, MD

 FINDHORN PRESS

Published in 2014 by Findhorn Press, Scotland

ISBN 978-1-84409-643-5

A CIP record for this title is available from the British Library.

Translated from the Spanish by Nick Inman
Edited by Nicky Leach
Front cover design and illustrations by Richard Crookes
Front cover photograph by Ksenia Kalinina
Interior design by Damian Keenan
Printed in the EU

Published by

Findhorn Press

117-121 High Street,

Forres IV36 1AB,

Scotland, UK

*t* +44 (0)1309 690582

*f* +44 (0)131 777 2711

*e* info@findhornpress.com

www.findhornpress.com

# CONTENTS

*To the wisdom of nature*

# Acknowledgments

Some years ago, I took part in a medical conference in Biarritz, France. On the last night, during a magnificent gala dinner, I found myself sitting around a large table with eight colleagues and friends—all of us doctors, scientists, and business people from different countries who had known each other for some time. After coffee was served, we sat a while in silence, thoughtful but close in spirit, then suddenly we began to play a "game," one that consisted of talking about our dreams and how we saw ourselves in 10 years' time. What did each of us hope to become, and what would we like to be doing for a living?

We allowed ourselves to be carried away by our dreams in complete freedom. It was a very tender and beautiful moment—a very rare experience for this group of mature people used to the world of business and routine. Why not, we thought? Tomorrow we would take our planes home, back to our responsibilities, but tonight we could allow ourselves the luxury of being open and sincere. The magic affected us all.

Each of us sat for a moment, with eyes closed and a gentle smile on the lips. Then, one by one, we listened to the inspiring stories of each person at the table, and the fantasies and dreams that he or she wanted to make a reality over the next decade.

I closed my eyes and allowed my imagination and my most intimate thoughts to fly freely. When it came to my turn to speak, I let myself go for the first time in my life and said aloud that I wanted to be a writer. I could imagine myself writing a book with great enthusiasm and professional pleasure. I saw myself in a very light place, in the sunshine, hearing the sound of the sea. I could visualize large windows and white curtains. I felt a sensation of fullness and satisfaction infusing my work and life. This dream seemed just that, though—an impossible and distant dream.

Now, all these years later, I offer you my first book. The original version was written in Spanish, a language that I did not know when I was at that conference in Biarritz, and never expected to learn, and here it has been translated into English. Today I live in Spain, even though at the time I could not have imagined in my wildest dreams that I would move from Prague to Madrid. Right now, I am looking at the Sierra de Madrid through large windows bordered by white curtains. I can't hear the sea, but I love this place where I now live.

I would like to share with you this magical transformation that I have had the privilege to live through in my normally busy and unpredictable life. I could never have imagined that the dreams I spoke of on that night spent with friends in Biarritz in 1999 would come true. Perhaps my desire to change was so intense that in the heat of the moment I made my choices and set my priorities without being aware of it.

I would like to say thank you especially to Mónica Liberman of the publishers La Esfera de los Libros, and to my Spanish editor Daniel Chumillas for his confidence and great patience. He believed in my project and gave this book a chance.

I would also like to thank some other important people: Carlos, my partner and teacher, without whom I would not be where I am; Vlad, my son and supporter, who motivates me to grow, to learn, and to keep abreast of the modern world; and my patient and wise mother, so committed to the family.

I owe gratitude, too, to all the teachers I have had, who at different times and in their distinct ways appeared in my path and shared their wisdom with me: my special master of medicinal plants, Carlos Andrin; my mentor and excellent therapist, Daniel Chumillas; the solitary philosopher Gustavo Muñoz; Jesús Valverde, friend and wise doctor; Darina Blahova, who breathes life in deeply and appreciates every moment of it; Andrei Matveikov, who helped me and supported me during a quantitative leap, both personal and work-related; Dr. Santiago de la Rosa for professional support; to my literary agent Elizabeth Wiggins for her great support and help; and to many, many more people.

I want to also thank my patients—many now friends—who accepted me with open arms and much curiosity and placed their confidence in me. They have helped me greatly and co-operated with me. In particular, I must thank those who have given me their testimonies in such a generous way: Yuyi Beringola, for the foreword; Teresa Bueyes; Joana Bonet; Miguel Ángel Solá; Rosa de la Torre; Dr. Ana María Ruiz Sancho; Dr. José Hernández Maraver; José Antonio Hernández Martín; Dr. Luis Bril; Pablo Pinilla; Paula Martínez; and those others who prefer to remain anonymous.

Finally, of course, I must express my gratitude to the rebelliousness of my own digestive system, which stimulates me, encourages me, and motivates me to continue learning about this hidden but intelligent being found in our gut.

# Foreword

When I was 12 years old, family problems made me very depressed, and I started to have terrible stomach pains. I was diagnosed with the beginnings of a duodenal ulcer, and I was put on a diet that I have mostly kept to ever since.

When I was 15, I lost my biological father, my marks at school went down from very good to just average, and then I started to have biliary colic pain, which left me feeling like a wreck. So I have absolutely no doubt that emotion and digestion are very closely related to each other.

After these colic episodes I was diagnosed with a "lazy" gallbladder, and the doctors told me that I also had a very sluggish liver. These are obviously things that don't show up on an ultrasound scan and at first sight don't seem too serious, but it is certainly true that all my life I have suffered from severe headaches, sometimes with such terrible nausea that I can't eat anything for weeks on end.

I work in the film business as a script supervisor and love my job, but it is not exactly the best thing for my digestion—irregular hours, filming at night for weeks on end; sometimes it's too hot, other times it's too cold; far too much traveling . . . but I've always tried to look after myself as best I can. My colleagues joke about me sometimes and say that I'm going to live forever like that, but that's not my aim. What I want is to live *well*. By that I mean enjoying my job and my life for as long as I can.

Perhaps I am aware of the importance of looking after myself because of my mother's story. She was a marvelous woman, full of energy, but she never took much care of herself and, at the age of 75, she had an intestinal obstruction, the result of chronic constipation, and had to have an emergency operation. She then had to have a second operation two years later, because something had come loose. Before these two operations I remember how she was the very last to leave the reception at my brother's wedding. Afterwards, she was never the same again.

Almost everyone has had some sort of problem with eating and food: some people lose their appetite for a time when they fall in love and can't eat anything; others can't stop eating when they have a problem, even though they know it won't agree with them.

A few years ago I read in a magazine that the legendary Swedish film director Ingmar Bergman always used to have diarrhea before the first day's filming. I understood him perfectly! The same thing had been happening to me all my life. Sometimes days would go by and I wouldn't feel like eating anything, and my friends would tell me: "How lucky you are, you're so slim!" But when I felt like eating again, I was so happy! I think that when you are healthy and full of life you feel hungry, too. It's a marvelous feeling.

Many Eastern philosophies talk about the body as the "temple" or the "vehicle"; in both cases they are referring to the importance of looking after our body and keeping it healthy and clean, because if we are not in good health, everything else becomes much more difficult.

Life is wonderful, but often we don't appreciate it. We are so busy with what is going on inside our head that we forget how to live and be present. We pay even less attention to what is happening inside our body; it's as if we are living disconnected from it and only think about it when something hurts. But sometimes that's already too late.

I started going to Irina's clinic quite recently. I had heard that she offered the liver and gall bladder therapy I wanted, which I was afraid to embark on by myself. She seemed splendid, so professionally committed but very kind at the same time, and she explained everything so clearly. She gave me an appointment for colonic hydro-therapy, something I had already had before but which I hadn't found at all pleasant; but anyhow, I thought, it has to be done. So early one morning I went along. To my surprise, Irina manages to make it all a pleasant experience. Her clinic is wonderful: it's full of energy and so bright and attractive. You can see that every last detail has been carefully thought out.

When the hydrotherapy was finished, she offered me a cup of herbal tea, and just that small detail changed everything—not the tea itself, although it was delicious, but the fact that she bothered to make it for me.

Irina is everything I expect in a doctor: someone who listens and explains things at your level and best of all, doesn't rush you.

I had my liver and gallbladder cleaned out, and it turned out to be more like a quarry than a liver: hundreds of stones came out! How could my poor liver possibly work properly with all that inside it? Since then, I've been back several times. Stones keep appearing, but at least I know I'm on the right track now, and I feel so much better.

Now when I have a headache I give myself a coffee enema, and most times it works. What a relief!

I believe that lots of things that happen to us can be cured by natural means, and this is something Irina does very well. I hope this book helps us all to get to know ourselves better and to understand what is happening to us, and that it encourages us to solve our problems.

— *YUYI BERINGOLA*, *FILM ACTRESS AND SCRIPTWRITER*

# Preface

The other day my bank branch manager (who also happens to be an obedient patient of mine) remarked: "I could never have been a doctor! You have too much responsibility for the health and life of others: I would feel dreadful. In the bank I can do something wrong, make an error, and nothing happens that I can't put right, but with the health of a human you can't make too many mistakes."

Modern society demands much of a doctor. We want to have the brilliant Dr. House as our GP and to stay in good health with a minimum of visits to the doctor's office, without taking pills and without suffering discomfort or pain.

Working in a bank you comply with financial regulations and the orders you are given, which leaves little room for any doubts; you do what you are asked to do, day after day. A visit to the doctor, however, is optional, not obligatory: you can postpone your checkups and ignore your problems if you want, and you can find fault with your practitioner and not follow her instructions.

Society doesn't force you to take care of yourself and to stay in good health. The most it does is to suggest and advise, but nobody makes sure that you are fit and well. It's not like that with bills and bank statements. To your bank manager, you are transparent and the diagnostic is always clear. To your doctor, you are a tired and secretive person with a series of problems that not even she knows how to begin to deal with. Are you going to listen to her and carry out her orders?

To stay in good health and prevent the development or advance of disease is your prerogative, but if you don't choose this course society won't cast you out. On the contrary, it will look after you as best it can—even if you think the care you are given is not sufficient. In Europe and most other western countries, when you fall ill, medical attention and hospital treatment will be provided. Your bank, on the other hand, will throw you out and close your account. At a medical health center, though, that is not our way; we are there to help you.

When you go to your bank, you are prepared and are already informed about the subject in hand. There is no reason why you cannot do the same when you come in for a medical consultation. Experts say that 80 percent of the care that a chronically ill person needs can be provided by himself, if he is given adequate preparation and training. They also estimate that 90 percent of the illnesses and problems that cause people to visit doctors could be prevented by following a healthy diet, doing a minimum of physical activity, and observing basic hygiene.

For doctors to be precise in their work and able to help their patients, they need enough space in their busy schedules for those 10 percent of cases that really need serious assistance. If the remaining 90 percent could be educated about health and personal care, imagine how helpful that would be.

Complaining about doctors, the health system and long waiting lists for tests only leads to anxiety and frustration, and in the short term will not improve things. So why not take another approach and get to know yourself?

Your body is your vehicle. It needs to be checked for roadworthiness; it needs good fuel; and it needs to be properly treated. To know your problems and take care of your health should be as essential as working or having a bank account. We should give the same importance to preventing ill health as we do to preventing bankruptcy.

Our health can and should be of interest to us. The purpose of this book is to encourage you to rise to the challenge of taking small but constant steps toward a healthy lifestyle—to discover your own "digestive intelligence."

The first thing to say is that we all have a second "brain," one that lies hidden deep inside our gut—a honed and powerful intelligence at our core, in the center of our bodies. It may seem strange, but it is important that we work with this intelligence, so that we can learn how to decipher the messages it sends us. My aim is to introduce you to the pleasure of recognizing, learning about, and respecting your digestive system—that marvelous and powerful being that occupies almost all the space inside you. Whether you make it a friend who helps and serves you or you mistreat it daily is your decision.

Treated well, the digestive system knows how to repair itself. It will start showing its appreciation for any positive changes you make within 15 hours, including changing to a better diet or giving it the care it needs. Yes, it's true that the same system can put up with months and years of mistreatment without complaining much, but if you want to have a good quality of life it is important to have good digestion.

This book does not replace your doctor or a visit to her surgery, if you really need one. Its aim is to provide you with a basic, up-to-date understanding of your digestive system, so that you can help your doctor to diagnose your problems. If you do this, you will give her the pleasure of communicating with an intelligent patient who knows how to be precise in his complaints and who applies the basic preventive measures in his daily life.

I favor an integrated, holistic style of medicine, which combines the advances of modern medicine with the wisdom of complementary forms of medicine, along with preventive measures. You have to treat the patient not the illness—to search for the root of the problem, not just patch up the symptoms.

Holistic medicine involves, primarily, the application of natural and less damaging methods of treatment to correct and coordinate the functions of all the body's systems. From day one, successful holistic treatment requires introducing changes in nutrition and hygiene and reeducating the patient about how their body works best. At the same time, however, holistic doctors work within the sphere of conventional medicine, and stay up to date on the latest medical knowledge, so that they can make accurate diagnosis of disease and choose the appropriate allopathic treatments involving drugs or equipment, if required. This skilled combination of allopathic and complementary modalities is the medicine of the future.

Unfortunately, a wide gulf still exists between mainstream medical professionals (those working in a public hospital or health center, for example) and naturopathic doctors. Frequently one denies the validity of the other—or doesn't have the time or will to try to understand anything outside the area of her professional interest. I do not take an extreme view on this, as I like to work with both kinds of medicine. This is why I feel that we must change this situation.

Twenty years ago, it was not my aim to specialize in gut health. I could not have imagined then that my work would one day consist of digging into the digestive problems of my patients and applying holistic principles of detoxification to treat them. As a young and perfectionist doctor, I wanted to save the world and treat the most serious patients, and I did this for some time. Toward the end of that part of my career, I dreamed of becoming a heart surgeon and literally "lived" next to the operating theater in order to gain experience.

The birth of my son turned everything upside down, however, and I found myself specializing in endocrinology, instead. I was lucky to be taught by specialists in that field who were associated with a leading center for the treatment of patients with complications arising from diabetes and other hormonal dysfunctions. It was work that never ended; a constant sacrifice and a permanent struggle with the patients. I was passionate about it.

To work like that 24 hours a day, seven days a week, is a way of not existing. You don't even notice the needs and requirements of your own body until you are worn out, and your family along with you. I began to feel physically unwell, and my digestive system declared war on me. I had to choose between my health and my career. My son, who was still young at the time, helped me to reach a decision. I switched to a less stressful job seeing outpatients, and it was there that I discovered that the patients we saved in emergencies were subsequently abandoned to their own devices. They did not know how to manage their illnesses or stick to guidelines. To make progress in this work and to help myself grow, I began to study different types of medicine.

I was fortunate to work in the pharmaceutical industry for many years, which enabled me to participate in clinical trials and attend important conferences, primarily related to oncology. I discovered another world: modern scientific medicine and cancer. For years we discussed the procedures of chemotherapy and radiotherapy, and the details of how to combat cancer. I have seen all sides of this tricky and, unfortunately, "very clever" illness. I have also had direct experience of it through close family members.

The circumstances of my life meant that I had to travel a great deal, and I took advantage of my visits to other countries to seek out the most authentic sources and the most distinguished teachers so that I could learn about natural and complementary medicines. This balanced my conventional professional work and gave me hope that one day I would be able to combine my experiences and apply my knowledge.

I believe that day has arrived.

> *Life teaches me that you feel and think as your digestion decides. To listen to Irina and read her words is an opportunity to think and feel better. Irina knows.*
> *A lot.*

— *MIGUEL ANGEL SOLA*, ACTOR

# 1

# Your Second Brain

Sometimes people joke about there being two brains: a female one inside the head and a male one inside the trousers. (The same comparisons are made of women's and men's hearts, too). If you think that in this chapter I'm going to talk about this supposed second brain—the pride and vanity hidden inside underwear—then you're mistaken. Although I do understand why that kind of "brain" is famous: its decision-making power is so strong that it isn't affected by the mental filters of cool rationality, common sense, and logic.

What I'm going to talk about in this book is another brain—the one inside our digestive system. It is not as glamorous and as interesting as our sex drive but can be just as wild and unpredictable—and we use it far more because our "digestive brain" goes into action several times every day.

It's fair to say that the intestine, which is divided into the large intestine and small intestine, is not the part of our anatomy we are most passionate about, nor the one that increases our pulse rate. No famous poet has written an ode to it, and normally artists are not inspired by the "beauty" of the digestive system. Quite the opposite, in fact. The most common view of the gut is that it is an ugly body part that looks a bit like a snake, smells bad, and sometimes makes socially unacceptable and embarrassing noises.

However, I promise you that we have a true second brain in our insides and its neuronal function is very similar to the brain in our heads. Inside our bellies there is an extensive network of neurons located between the two muscular layers of the walls of the digestive system. Moreover, the structure of these digestive neurons is identical to that of neurons in the brain: both produce similar chemical molecules—neurotransmitters and hormones that are mostly necessary for our intercellular communications and the correct functioning of the body.

Let me introduce you to the enteric nervous system (ENS), our "second brain." This is not a metaphor; it is the official name accepted by medical professionals. The importance of the ENS was only demonstrated relatively recently with the publication of the work of Professor Michael Gershon, chairman of the Department of Anatomy and Cell Biology at Columbia University, New York, and the forerunner of the new science of *neurogastroenterology*. This new area of speciality studies the symptoms of psychosomatic upsets that have a gastrointestinal expression and relates them to the central nervous system (CNS). Dr. Gershon has spent 30 years of his scientific career on an in-depth study of the attitude and behavior of the human gut, and he has confirmed that our nervous digestion system has its own cerebral activity and intelligence. His book, *The Second Brain: A Groundbreaking New Understanding of Nervous Disorders of the Stomach and Intestine* (Gershon, 1999), was a significant step forward in information on the ENS, advancing the existing medical and scientific understanding of the subject.

According to new data, the total number of neurons found in the small intestine is around a hundred million. This figure represents a considerably higher number of neurons than in the spinal cord, for example. The brain in our gut is the main production line responsible for producing and storing the chemical substances called *neurotransmitters,* most of which are identical to those found in the central nervous system (CNS), such as *acetylcholine, dopamine* and *serotonin.* These substances regulate our moods and our emotional and psychological well-being. They form a group of essential substances ensuring correct communication between the neurons and the body's warning system. They represent the "words" in the neuronal language. The presence of such a wide variety of neurotransmitters in our intestines is a clear indication of the complexity of the rich digestive language and its ability to carry out neuronal functions and express its own emotions.

Gershon revealed that 90 percent of serotonin (the famous "happiness" or "feel-good" hormone ) is produced and stored in the intestinal walls, where it regulates peristaltic movements and sensory transmission. Only the remaining 10 percent of the body's serotonin is synthesized in the neurons of the central nervous system—the brain, or our "higher brain." The minimum amount of serotonin in the higher brain is, nevertheless, of vital importance for human beings. It performs various functions, including regulating our mood (the calm "feel-good" sensation), appetite, sleep, and muscular contractions, and it intervenes in cognitive functions such as  memory and learning. Serotonin is the "messenger of happiness," and thanks to it the neurons can communicate with each other, releasing it and capturing it again as needed.

Before this revelation, the scientific world did not pay much attention to this aspect of the intestines and did not appreciate the nerve network that runs through them. The general view was that the decisions made by the higher brain were dominant and that its influence on the digestive system was one way, that is, the process was directed downward from the central nervous system. The scientific observations made by Professor Gershon, however, now lead us to think that influence travels in both directions—that there is constant communication between the two brains: the one inside our skull and its brother down there in our gut.

I can assure you that the relationship between the two brains, which involves hormonal, metabolic, and emotional levels, is very complex—we could even call it "intellectual"; it is also normally quite democratic and mutually respectful.

## Curious Facts about Evolution

Evolution is magical. Millions of years ago, when our ancestors were developing their spinal column and the basic structures of the cranial brain were just starting to appear, they already had a nervous system in their gut, which allowed them to survive and evolve.

This ancient brain was in charge of all the vital visceral functions and was completely independent and well coordinated. Our forebears were already able to spend more time and energy on the important and enjoyable activities of life—building up experience, defending themselves, and indulging in sexual behavior—while their intestinal brain took charge of their nutrition, digestion, absorption, hydration, and elimination of waste matter.

In the earliest developments of the cerebral cortex, the mental activity of our ancestors was more basic than ours today; it was guided more by instinct and intuition. In other words, our distant relatives listened to their guts and acted on the signals their intestinal brains sent them. For animals, in fact, the voice of the "enteric" brain is still the predominant communicator of information. We are often amazed at the accuracy of a dog, horse, or cat's intuition. Animals pay attention to the signals coming from their innards. We "higher beings," in contrast, are now separate from the rest of the animal world (although not completely), and we have suppressed the intuitive capacity associated with a "gut feeling," in favor of the all-powerful guiding voice of our mind and conscience.

Nevertheless, each of us from time to time has a "gut feeling," a warning that comes from deep inside and appears in intense or extreme emotional situations. It presents itself as a whole range of sensations, from a pleasurable thrill to a nervous knot, a hollow feeling, or a pain. This is our intestinal brain talking to us. Poor brain. To attract our attention and goad us into action, it has to shout loudly using its own "language": bouts of diarrhea, spasms, or nausea.

The intestinal brain has developed alongside its higher twin, growing in size, and increasing the diversity and quantity of neurochemical substances produced. It has perfected its control of the vital functions and adapted to the new demands and needs of the human body. This evolution continues today. Apart from the tasks mentioned above, its work consists in assimilating information about new chemical substances that pass through its digestive "border control."

After prolonged development, the enteric nervous system has been transformed into something much more important than a mere relic of our ancestors: it is now a modern system that performs highly complex vital functions without us having to make any mental effort or control its work.

## Out of Control

There's no way we can control our digestive functions with our minds. Imagine if we could dictate: "Today I'm not going to need a laxative to go to the toilet." Or "the roast lamb I'm going to eat today at my mother-in-law's is going to agree with me very well." That's not how it is. Our powerful mental control stops the moment we start eating and starts again at the end of evacuation. We are aware of the two orifices at either end of the digestive system, which have completely opposed functions. It's only logical! The mind can be cunning and deceitful, and the decisions we make sometimes don't make sense. Nature can't allow us to manipulate our nutritive, digestive, and immunological functions according to our consciences or let them be the victims of our unpredictable moods. We wouldn't have been able to survive that way.

It's strange, isn't it? With willpower and intelligence we can change the world, yet we can't change our own digestion—or even influence it—without specialized knowledge. This enrages some people. The power that their own digestive system has over them makes them cross; they just can't accept this internal rebellion, which doesn't fit into their day-to-day agenda. But not everything is under our mental control—and that includes our digestion. What we have to do is to sign a pact, to enter into a diplomatic relationship with our gut, so that it collaborates with us and lets us get on with our lives.

I often see this anger and lack of patience in my patients. They expect to improve their digestion, reduce their bloating, and cure their constipation or their irritable colon by exerting pressure; it's almost as if they are making a demand on their bodies and on their doctor—something has to be achieved and as soon as possible. If in two weeks' time it seems like "nothing is working" and they don't see any "magic" change, then they get frustrated.

The intestinal brain, however, does not agree to any old compromise. It requires long-term treatment and care until it recovers its health and internal balance. Just as we can't cure anxiety and depression in a couple of weeks, we can't treat digestive neurosis in a few days, either.

People who come looking for alternative help with their digestive system normally bring problems with them that have been dogging them for years, and they are desperate. I often wonder why their reaction to the prospect of a few months' work on their intestines and their diet is, "Oh no, that's too much."

## Caring for Yourself with Complementary Medicine is Back in Fashion

At last! It doesn't surprise me in the least that nowadays people are showing a renewed interest in alternative and complementary medications, shamanism, native rituals, meditation techniques, and other ways to reconnect with their own bodies. The ancient idea of *mindfulness* has come back into fashion. We are attracted by the concepts of Buddhism. Spirituality is becoming increasingly important to us, and we feel the need to recontact nature and withdraw from the stress of everyday life. I consider this new evolutionary twist to be both beautiful and logical.

It is already becoming clear to many of us that stress, tension, never-ending work, and responsibilities exhaust the body and the mind and cause the systems of the body to start to fail—beginning with the digestive and psychological functions.

So what can we do? To stop the world and change our lives seems impossible. Medications don't seem to be the solution to everything, either. Current studies and research in biotechnology and modern neuroscience are very important and hold great promise for the medicine of the future, but it is early days yet in terms of their practical application.

In spite of everything, now more than ever the search for inner harmony and the use of complementary medicine and spiritual philosophies offer *real* steps that we can take in our daily lives. And they are within reach of everyone.

But let's go back to our two brains. Our brain capacity is much greater than we normally use. (Apparently, we usually only use around 15 percent of our brain's potential). We have the internal mechanisms we need for recovery and cure. Our body talks to us and warns us. If we could just decode its signals and take notice of them, we would be much stronger and healthier.

Like a good twin, the intestinal brain shares, takes responsibilty for, and assimilates the emotions and problems its higher brother generates, and records in the memory of our entrails those emotional events that have the strongest impact.

## Two-Way Emotional Influence

Here are some examples of how the upper brain influences our digestion and how our digestive behavior affects our thoughts and moods:

- A very tense emotional situation, or a state of terror or a traumatic event may make you vomit, or else provoke diarrhea or cause total indigestion.
- When you feel lonely, or frustrated sentimentally, or when your self-esteem has been destroyed, the psychological state you are in can influence your metabolism and the complex processes of digestion. This may cause lack of appetite, disgust, or indifference and a slow and troublesome digestion.

More often this "chronic unhappiness" is expressed as a state of anxiety and compulsive behavior, with uncontrollable binge eating at critical moments, usually mid-afternoon and late at night. This compulsive and uncontrolled eating (especially carbohydrates) leads to a rapid release of hormones and chemical substances in both brains which induce a temporary feeling of well-being and overall satisfaction. Shortly afterwards, however, this neuronal mechanism "runs out of steam," the digestion breaks down and heaviness and bloating develop; the digestive system starts to groan and protest at this food abuse and this is accompanied by a guilty feeling. Your self-esteem reaches its lowest ebb and you begin to regret what you have done. At this point, many women decide to make themselves vomit.

Let's follow with some more examples of how the two brains communicate with each other:

- A bout of diarrhea with episodes of colic and spasms (which may be the flaring-up of irritable bowel condition or gastroenteritis) prevents you from thinking clearly. It's as if your irritability and sensitivity are turned up to maximum volume and you feel overcome by tiredness and exhaustion. This makes you bad-tempered and lowers your level of intellectual productivity.
- Constipation accompanied by bloating makes you feel that your life is "weighing you down" with its problems (and your stomach feels the same) and you lose all interest in social and physical activities. You may not believe me but chronic constipation can turn a person into a sarcastic pessimist, lowering the libido and limiting his sex life. Whatever the reason for the constipation, it can lead to a lower level of serotonin (or a lower sensitivity to this hormone) produced by the neurons in the intestinal brain. This limits digestive muscular motility (the ability of the intestinal muscles to generate soft and regular movements and contractions, which mix and propel contents in the gastrointestinal tract) and this in turn triggers a lack of positive emotions. On the other hand, slow intestinal transit increases the toxic overload in our organism.
- A buildup of emotions in the guts is very common in women who are perfectionists and want to control everything; it's as if the control center of their lives were in their intestines. This attitude generates particularly serious constipation that is resistant to classic treatments and remedies.
- Some people suppress their emotions and they are unable to express themselves; they do not know how to show affection and so they often experience

an internal rebellion: episodes of profuse diarrhea, an irritable bowel, and oversensitized digestion.

- A good bowel movement in the morning, which leaves you feeling pleasantly light and clean, is a very good way to start the day. It puts you in a good mood, makes you feel full of energy and everything looks positive. I'm sure you agree.

- You wake up with a bad taste in your mouth, with no appetite and you can't face having breakfast, your insides having been bunged up for days. You are too busy thinking of other things to clear yourself out and you rush out after a quick cup of coffee. The day doesn't look very promising and certainly won't leave you feeling good since you are already emotionally prepared for it to be a thoroughly grey day.

Our two brains are both masters. They engage, talk, sabotage, or reinforce each other. It depends on the day and the emotional and digestive situation. What kind of day will you decide to have?

## The Enormous Hidden Potential of Your Gut

It has been shown that the digestive system has tremendous neurological and hormonal potential. This is why scientists and the pharmaceutical industry are currently devoting so much of their research and testing to neurogastroenterology.

The psychopharmacological medications prescribed on a massive scale for depression belong to the group of drugs called selective serotonin reuptake inhibitors (SSRIs). These drugs facilitate neuronal communication by prolonging the active presence of serotonin in the space between two neurons (the synapse, or synaptic gap, as mentioned earlier) before it is recaptured by the receptors. Such drugs have an effect on only 10 percent of cerebral serotonin—that which passes across the synaptic gap—and they are said to improve the patient's mood and control depression.

As we have discussed, our gut brain produces a sea of serotonin—the remaining 90 percent of this hormone associated with happiness and well-being. The question is, therefore: How can we take advantage of this valuable resource and make the best use of it for mental and digestive health? This is a challenging task for researchers. In addition, scientists have made the surprising finding that the gut is also a rich source of endogenous benzodiazepines, which are the active ingredient in anxiolytic drugs (tranquilizers). These are the drugs prescribed to help us sleep, overcome stress, reduce anxiety, or treat phobias. This raises the intriguing question: What if we could activate our own resources and somehow release digestive anxiolytics for our own psychoemotional needs? Nothing is impossible; we have all the solutions inside ourselves.

Have you noticed that a baby's tummy is particularly sensitive? When the mother or father massages it gently, the baby's digestion and problems with gas improve—the child calms down, stops crying, and goes to sleep more quickly. This effect is similar to that of endogenous benzodiazepines (produced inside the body) but is induced naturally. As adults we don't seem to find the time to love our intestines. We are just not used to massaging them or indulging in professional massages, and/or doing exercises to relax our abdomens. We shouldn't forget that the gentle therapeutic touch of hands always has a calming, relaxing effect, and can sometimes even be curative.

The opioid receptors (the cells in the brain that capture and reinforce the effect of substances such as morphine) are also found in the intestines. This explains the effect of morphine and heroin on the digestive system, since the second brain develops a dependence on these drugs just like the other brain.

If digestive upsets can cause insomnia or restless sleep patterns, the reverse is also true: insomnia or lack of rest and sleep (often because of stress or work problems ) can cause digestive upsets. The electroencephalographic (EEG) record, the evaluation of electric brain waves of the five phases of sleep, has an equivalent in the electromyographic (EMG) record, the evaluation of the electric waves of the intestinal muscles of the digestive nervous system, which has identical sleep cycles. Studies show that people with digestive problems also have abnormal REM (Rapid Eye Movement) sleep; this is the lightest sleep phase, essential for complete rest and memory assimilation.

I emphasize that there is a direct connection between the psyche and the stomach. Many intestinal problems can be explained by the malfunctioning of the "intestinal brain" or by interferences in its communication with the higher brain. The gut brain is where fear, anxiety, or phobias originate, along with excessive control or obsessions, and also premonition, apprehension, and intuition. Scientists consider that the abdominal brain can also memorize certain emotions, experience stress, and suffer its own psychoneurosis.

The famous phrase is "I think, therefore I am." To this we would now have to add "… if my gut lets me." Vomiting, diarrhea, and spasms all cloud the mind. The enteric nervous system would never write poetry or engage in a Socratic dialogue, but in spite of that, it really is a more intuitive brain, although without much social influence. In the words of Professor Michael Gershon: "The intestinal brain plays an important role in human happiness and misery, although few people even know they have one."

## The Digestive Brain Concept in Eastern Philosophies

Although Western medicine has only recognized the "second brain" recently, in Eastern medicine the belly has long been viewed as the vital center of the human organism. Traditional world medications and their treatises on the digestive system comprise an enormously wide-ranging subject, which perhaps merits a separate book; however, we can briefly mention here some of these philosophies to give just a taste of how authentic wisdom integrates the human being in all its aspects : physical, spiritual, and energetic.

Traditional Chinese medicine (TCM) recognizes the gut as the *dantian,* loosely translated as the "navel area, the center of energy, the sea of *qi.*" Qi is the vital energy, force, or impulse, similar to *prana* in Hinduism, *pneuma* in classical Greek, and *élan vital* in the term coined by the French philosopher Henri Bergson.

The Hindu tradition of healing locates the third of the seven *chakras,* or energy "wheels," in the same place as the intestinal brain. The third, or solar plexus, chakra *(manipura,* or "shining jewel"), is located in the middle of the torso, in the diaphragm area above the navel, at the body's center of gravity. This is where Universal Life is expressed as Existential Life; it is the center of the human being, body and soul. In contrast to the energy controled by willpower or "doing," the *qi* in the belly is "felt" and "allowed to come." Ideally, we should be in contact with this center (the gut itself) and concentrate its energy.

In Japanese martial arts, the *hara,* like the dantian above, represents "the belly, man's center of being, the sea of qi. " This is where the expression *hara kiri* comes from, traditionally a form of ritual suicide among samurai warriors but literally meaning "belly-cutting" or severing the energy of being.

To be "hara-centered" is equivalent to an optimal state of health and integration of all the bodily systems, longevity, and well-being. It leads to a general state of serenity and profound calm, awareness, reason, personal power, and balanced action. This state can be achieved through meditation and psychophysical disciplines, including tai chi, qigong (chi kung), or hatha yoga.

Those who have a well-developed hara can do many things without any apparent effort, while at the same time remaining calm, patient observers who do not feel the need to intervene, even if they are not in agreement. Those who know the art of hara *(haragei,* the "art of the stomach") are immediately conscious of when they leave the "just center" and fall under the influence of the egocentric self; and quite naturally, without any effort, they are able to return to their center. Those with weak hara have fragile health, get angry, and lose their temper easily; when faced with adversity, they quickly lose their self-control. The psychosomatic expression "to be centered," or in contact with our internal energy, has a lot to do with having a balanced digestive system in the language of Western medicine.

The body is a true treasure available to us, but it only works fully if we respect it and let it act as it needs to, without submitting it to external aggressions that knock it off balance.

*We live in the most narcissistic society in human history. Cultivating our image has become a social requirement, but we often forget our interior life. In our hygienic and aseptic society, which desperately seeks a high-quality lifestyle and maximum satisfaction, there is no sense in not looking inwards and being aware of our own bodies. This is why the work of professionals like Irina Matveikova, MD is essential, not just for her therapeutic contribution but also for her educational approach, showing us what we have chosen to ignore and encouraging us to embark on a healthier lifestyle, leading to a real sensation of well-being and vital hygiene.*

— *JOANA BONET*, DIRECTOR, MARIE CLAIRE MAGAZINE, WRITER AND JOURNALIST.

# 2

# The Virtues of the
# Digestive System

Welcome to the world of digestion! This is a good moment to begin to decipher the demands of your gut and to create a friendly relationship with your second brain.

The aim of this book is to describe the physiological, emotional, and intellectual potential that we have in our digestive systems, and to teach you to listen to, learn from, and work with your gut. To do this will not only bring purely digestive benefits but will also lead to physical, psychological, and emotional well-being. I invite you to take a trip through your digestive tract, with various stops at particular points of interest along the way.

The total length of the digestive tract is 8–12 meters (25–40 ft.). Were it to be straightened out it would reach the height of a two-story building. It is not only long but also wide. If you could imagine the total area of your intestines spread out flat in two dimensions it would cover 300 square meters (3000 sq. ft.). That means you have the equivalent area of a tennis court hidden in your gut!

Over a lifetime, approximately 70 tons of food and 100 tons of liquid pass through your digestive system. Your gut is able to process, analyze, absorb, and eliminate this industrial quantity without breakdowns or the need for replacement parts—if, that is, it is treated well. That is a big *if*, as we so often mistreat our digestive systems, even though they are alerting us to alterations in their normal functioning by sending us signals and warnings that they are in urgent need of "service."

The digestive system has a spectacular design. To give one example: the inner lining of the small intestine is "folded" into thousands of villi and on the surface of each of these are thousands of microvilli (smaller folds). Under a microscope, the lining of the small intestine looks like a dense brush or a piece of velvet fabric. These anatomical intricacies enable the mucosa to completely absorb all the vital nutrients in our food and exert immunological control—70 percent of the total immune defences of the body are found in the belly.

## Are We Hollow?

We are used to thinking of our bodies as solid, and that everything that lies beneath our skin belongs to an inside world. It would be more correct to say that we are hollow. The design of the human body is much more interesting and artistic than you may think.

Running through the middle of the body is a long tunnel, the digestive tract. The space inside this tunnel (the *lumen*, from the Latin for light or opening inside a tubular structure), bordered by the inner layers of the mucosa, carries substances that don't belong to you. This strange exterior world flows inside you, transporting foods, liquids, substances, chemicals, and bacteria—everything that you have swallowed and consumed. The digestive tract controls the passage of all these foreign substances, as they pass through your body from the mouth to the anus during digestion. En route, the foods you eat are assimilated and become the building blocks that make up your body; they become you.

The digestive mucosa is the body's customs service: a "high-intelligence service of the state." You depend on its work for your health and your life. The digestion and absorption of nutrients that it undertakes are vital functions, as essential as breathing and the beating of the heart. A bad digestion should be given equal importance to poor respiration or a cardiac condition.

Looked at in a certain way, you really are hollow. Your essence and continuity is interrupted by the lumen of this tube that runs through you carrying foreign substances; this tube is in charge of the vital functions of defence, strength, nutrition, energy, growth, construction of new tissues, and detoxification.

## Digestive Emotions

Your intestines have another virtue, too: the digestive system detects, processes, channels, and generates emotions. "We feel it in our gut" or "feel gutted." We "psychosomatize" emotions and stress. Through our gut, we have premonitions and intuitions, hide fears, and store childhood memories. If we receive good news we may notice a pleasant flutter in our belly. Conversely, a situation of tension or fear can tie a knot in our stomach or give us the sensation of a mouse gnawing at us. Emotional reactions can cause nausea, vomitting, diarrhea or, at the other extreme, block our digestion function.

As we have seen in the previous chapter, each of us has a digestive brain, or enteric nervous system, that has millions of neurons which, via multiple neurotransmitters, have the power to influence both our digestion and our psychological state.

## The Journey of a Slice of Chocolate Cake

This is a good moment to review human anatomy—in particular, the perfect design of our digestive system. Let's take the example of something special you like to eat, say a slice of chocolate cake for dessert, although it could be a steak or anything rich that you don't eat every day. When you think of a piece of cake, your central and peripheral nervous systems receive information about this imaginary meal and unleash multiple psychological reactions and enzymes associated with its possible digestion. Most notably, your mouth starts to water.

When the slice of cake reaches your stomach it has to share the space with whatever else you have eaten—salad, a main course, vegetables, wine, and so on. One kind of food bumps against another in your inner cauldron. Your stomach tells you that it is full and begins to grow beyond the limits of your belt. Simultaneously, the food you have eaten activates digestive neuronal processes that liberate hormones of well-being. Your body feels satisfied; it loosens up and relaxes. This puts you in a good mood, and you may feel the need to have a siesta or at least to sit down comfortably for a while.

Unfortunately, for many people, foods such as a rich dessert provoke multiple digestive discomforts after they have eaten them, even occasionally. However, we must be careful with our conclusions about the causes of these digestive limitations, because that tasty piece of cake shouldn't harm or bother anyone, and there is no need to blame it. It is the digestive system itself that has lost the capacity to adapt itself to different foods—to assimilate and process them well, in a speedy and healthy form.

To consciously limit the consumption of some foods, with the aim of looking after yourself, preventing illness, or as a decision in the interests of the environment, sounds logical and correct. But to remove chocolate cake or any other food forever from your life just because it causes stomachache, heartburn, or another complaint is a forced response to your discomfort, not a solution to it. Before accepting it as a perennial state, it is worth trying to correct the digestive response and to look for a healthy compromise. If you are not going to eat rich foods, it should be a deliberate decision of your brain not the result of digestive suffering.

To put a rich morsel in your mouth, then chew it and swallow it is the last conscious act that you make in the entire digestive process; the rest is beyond your control or awareness. When you swallow a mouthful of food, you lose touch with what happens to it inside the digestive tract. You only become aware of it again at the other end, when you expel the remains. Without mental control or additional force on your part, the cake will end up becoming blood, muscles, energy, and essential nutrients, and the residue will leave in the form of feces.

The digestive system is an extraordinary being that thinks for you without involving the brain, repairs damage, and puts up with the maltreatment that you give it. We do not, in general, appreciate any of this enough. All that you are likely to know about it are sensations: the signals that are sent by your digestive brain.

For example, after eating you may feel good; you may be relaxed, in a good mood, and content with everything because your gut is sending you a feeling of well-being. But the opposite can happen. You can instead feel full, heavy, and bloated; you can experience reflux, heartburn, and drowsiness, and this can put you in a bad mood.

The poor cake can repeat on you for several hours, leaving a bad taste in your mouth and impeding your digestion. Suddenly, your clothes feel tight and your thresholds of irritation and frustration are lowered. The same kind of food can be experienced in very different ways by different people: one may associate it with the tedium of obligatory family meals accompanied by tension, while another may regard it as opportunity for the pleasure of sharing a meal in good company. You choose. How? By getting to know the personality of your digestive system.

## Is There Such a Thing as "Delicate" Digestion?

I want to ask you to abandon this notion of "delicate digestion," when there is no physiological or pathological reason for it. By believing in digestive delicacy, or sensitivity, as if it were karma, you not only sacrifice many important foods but by convincing yourself to eliminate them permanently from your diet in favor of eating in a bland and monotonous way, you also run the risk of creating nutritional deficiencies. Placing gastronomic limits on yourself also prevents you from enjoying a meal with workmates or with your family; this in itself can affect your psychoemotional state.

If you can't eat a cake or a steak from time to time (not too often and not in excess, of course), it indicates that your system is suffering from a provisional upset, an error in your programming. This breakdown can be diagnosed, and you can learn to control it.

Appearance, sex, race, age, or occupation do not make any difference to our ability to eat well and to digest well—as long as we are talking about healthy eating. Delicate, slim, sensitive people with discerning and intellectual dispositions, and strong, stout almost brutish people: all of us are capable (that is, we are designed and programmed) to eat everything, cake and steak included, and to experience a normal digestion. There is a myth of inner fragility and many people think that they have weak stomachs and accept this, without looking for reasons as to why this should be.

Each person simply needs to understand the style and character of his own digestion, to match his meals to his energetic needs and daily activities, and then to balance the quality and quantity of dishes eaten. You can train your digestive system to carry out its functions regularly and completely, and to tolerate a variety of foods.

We all enter this world as babies, and from infancy we gradually develop conditioned reflexes that will, over time, come to define our digestive systems and their capacities. A baby cries when it is hungry, expels its waste products regularly without warning, and sleeps a lot. We love all this: it seems natural and magical. We teach children little by little to eat at set mealtimes and to use the toilet; we also regulate their times for sleep and activity. The process is not always easy, and it obviously requires time, because we begin at zero. However, if we apply our teaching methods with love and patience, a child of three is able to manage its own hunger and last until the next mealtime, to sleep through the night, and to understand the purpose of a toilet.

We feed children progressively, according to their needs, increasing the diversity of the foods we offer them and the variety of textures; their mucosas adapt perfectly to the changes and learn to process and benefit from all they eat. Each child lives through a transformation in his digestive system from basic, intuitive instincts and a sterile inner environment to a learned and conditioned behavior of his guts (varying according to his family circumstances and the society and culture he lives in). He thus acquires an intestinal microflora that will serve him all his life. As he goes through childhood and adult life, there will inevitably be various factors that influence his digestion negatively and temporarily, but his digestive system will never lose the capacity to learn, be trained, and educated.

If you want to be master of your body, in control of your digestion, it may be necessary to begin at zero, deploying patience and constancy, preferably with the aid of professional assessment and supervision. You probably won't have to wait three years like a child to regain good digestive reflexes, but you will certainly have to give it your full attention and dedicate several months to your digestion, your emotions, and your diet.

It will be worth it! I encourage you not to give up—not to give in to medications and limitations, but rather to undertake a complete work of digestive and dietary education.

Sometimes it is best to begin on your journey toward having a healthy and intelligent digestion with a digestive cleaning and detoxification and a strictly reduced, body-purifying diet. In my clinic we call this "fine tuning the digestive system." We regard it as a kind of internal vehicle inspection and service that reveals problems and helps the patient accept the need for change and to motivate himself.

* * * * * * * *

C. is a young, tall, and slim opera singer. Because of the character of her metabolism, her hormonal profile, and her energetic needs, she eats like a horse. She doesn't let a day go by without eating a generous portion of varied proteins, pulses, vegetables, and some cereals. Her body, visibly fragile and delicate, demands "combustibles" in quality and quantity.

She has learned how to divide her daily diet into five meals and chew well. She has developed new tastes and has ceased to be devoted to carbohydrates and desserts.

Today, C. doesn't have any digestive troubles. She has an extraordinary voice and, of course, wants to become a star. She knows that her talent has to be nourished and supported by good health. Few people are as aware as her!

C. has learned to listen to the warnings of her insides and to not ignore them. To restore her digestion, she immediately undertook a diet lasting 3–5 days, based on varied foods that were all liquidized, steamed, or boiled and served in the form of soups and purées (the same as little children often eat). As well as this, she was advised to drink a lot of hot medicinal herb teas to help her digestion, taking her thermos flask with her to the opera house.

Other good tips are to take a hot bath with salts in the evening (soaking for 20–30 minutes), and to go to bed with a blanket to relax the guts and help calm intestinal spasms. The digestive system doesn't need much before it will thank you for it and work well.

It is a simple case history but with a moral. If you have a relationship with your digestive brain based on a misunderstanding and misinterpretation and it starts to rebel and require attention, pay it heed (as in any relationship it is better to take action sooner rather than later), and in a few days you will be back in charge of your health and you will understand your digestion.

* * * * * * * *

Another of my patients is a sportsman who has a perfect body, but a digestive system totally damaged by the continual consumption of artificial supplements that contain too many proteins and hormones. He doesn't eat balanced, carefully made meals rich in fiber and nutrients. His principal complaints are lack of appetite, energy, and enthusiasm; inability to concentrate on his work; and bloating and constipation. His belly is swollen and prominent, and this frustrates him.

If you saw this man you would not describe him as delicate: he is the very definition of physical force. However, he has managed to acquire a delicate, unbalanced digestion and an irritable intestine. He needed to be put on a strict diet: light and very different from his previous one. I hope I can make him aware of the needs of his body and convince him to make important changes to his lifestyle, and to have patience.

The moral of this story is that sport does not forgive bad eating habits and cannot be a substitute for them. Not everything in life is achieved through force of will and muscle. Victory is no use if you jeopardize your health and energy in pursuit of it. You can't skip the fundamental rules of good nutrition and correct digestion without reaping dire consequences.

I repeat that, in origin, we are perfect in design. The body is programmed to be adaptable and to do its work well, processing varied foods when they are consumed in reasonable quantities. It is a powerful system, capable of recovering and adjusting its enzyme functions to its needs, as well as regenerating its mucosa and recovering its balance, in spite of the alimentary upheavals perpetrated on it by its owner.

My professional objective is to show you that if you deliberately eliminate one element from your diet with the aim of solving a regular digestive problem, you have to try to reintroduce it as an option later, without fear or complications, so that it doesn't become "forbidden fruit" forever. I want you to be able to say, "I can eat it, but I choose not to because it is not healthy" or "I don't have a great craving for that, but if I ate it I would feel great, without any upset or regret."

Some of my patients who are now in the maintenance phase of their digestive health, tell me that now and then they get a craving to "try something bad," something they haven't eaten for a long time. They want to "push the boundaries" of their restored digestive systems to see how far they can go. One of them, for example, decides to eat a steak; another goes to a burger and fries fast food restaurant with his children; and a third goes out for drinks "in style." All of them are surprised by the tolerant and healthy response of their guts after the fact, as if nothing had happened, and this reminds them a lot of their youth. It is very satisfying to know that you can "go over the top" on the odd occasion, and that the digestive system will cope, but I beg you to do it only on the odd occasion, and briefly, and afterwards to reestablish your previous balance.

It is a euphoric sensation not to feel bad, to allow yourself to do something suppressed and forbidden, and not have to suffer for it. Normally, if you go "over the top" once only, things calm down afterwards, the craving is satisfied, and the case is closed. "I can do it," you conclude, "but my health is more important to me, and I don't want to try it again, now that I have a more selective and exquisite taste."

Food is a pleasure and fun. It's worth keeping it that way. To sign a peaceful agreement with your digestive system and set up a system of diplomatic cooperation makes good sense.

*My life has always been marked by the competition and hyperactivity of the music business. Discovering and launching groups, the pressure to produce hits, the search for that song which will be a success, stress and more stress ...*

*mealtimes disrupted, travel, changing city and country, jet lag—these have all taken a toll on my health and my mood.*

*My consultation with Dr. Irina and her advice to improve my daily dietary habits, and at the same time cleaning my insides with sessions of hydrotherapy, have brought me great benefits, both mentally and emotionally.*

*To eat well, at suitable times and, above all, to know the foods that your body tolerates well, and to "clean out the pipes" of your digestive system a couple of times a year is the best advice to follow at any age.*

*Thank you, Irina, for showing me how to practice "intelligent digestion."*

— **PABLO PINILLA**, MUSIC PRODUCER

3

# Emotion and Digestion – Irritable Bowel Syndrome

*It is much more important to know what sort of a patient has a disease than what sort of a disease a patient has.*

— WILLIAM OSLER

· · · · · · · · ·

L., 53 years old, thinks of himself as a healthy person except for inherited hypercholesterolaemia (high cholesterol caused by a genetic condition), which he manages with medication. L, however, has symptoms compatible with an irritable bowel syndrome. He is a professional who is passionate about his work: a little stressed, obsessive, and neurotic, although he is charming and takes charge of everything. His personality is that of speedy control freak—obsessive and perfectionist—which is very typical of someone with irritable bowel syndrome.

A very good friend decided that L. needed help after a curious incident. One day the two of them were in his office to deal with various unpleasant work issues. At a critical point of the discussion, L. became exaggeratedly emotional, communicating this in a passionate form with expressive body language. In this moment, an unexpected sneeze unleashed an irreversible chain of events. Almost instantaneously, accompanied by an orchestral sound, L.´s guts expelled all of their warm and liquid contents!

L.´s guts bubbled and rumbled while his underwear and trousers became saturated with a suspicious damp. This prevented him from making brusque movements. He didn't dare leave the room screaming, to disappear, to evaporate. Instead, he froze in his chair, becoming soaked in the "broth".

It wasn't long before a treacherous stench began to fill the air of the office: it was a foul-smelling, asphyxiating gas that stung the eyes and provoked retching.

The silence between the two colleagues seemed to last an eternity. Confused and disoriented, neither knew what to do. The sound of the telephone broke the ice, and the two began to react, L. excusing himself with all the words he could think of, while his colleague tried to console him and help by offering a box of Kleenex and a packet of moist towels for removing makeup.

They managed to get L. to the toilets located in the corridor without encountering anyone who would be a witness and without dropping telltale drops on the floor.

Once locked in the toilet, L. had to wait a long time while his colleague bought him a new pair of trousers in a nearby shop. All traces of the crime were cleared up. Their friendship proved solid, because no one ever found out what had occurred, and the two continued working together as if nothing had happened.

This is a an example of the "triumphal" appearance of irritable bowel syndrome in full manifestation. Nevertheless, L. took his time in calling me and making an appointment: he waited until his rebellious intestines were on the verge of a new French Revolution.

He arrived in my consulting room with a report from a recent visit to a hospital emergency room indicating that the patient had presented with a strong retroesternal pain (in the chest, behind the sternum) that they suspected had its origin in the heart. Considering his medical history, the doctors carried out some rapid checks and concluded that it was an acute outbreak of irritable bowel syndrome without any other pathology. An x-ray showed an excessive buildup of feces and gas throughout his intestinal tract. The distension of the colon was especially pronounced in the upper left part (in the splenic flexure of the colon), and this had provoked discomfort and pains similar to a heart attack.

Fortunately, L. stuck rigorously to all the treatment and advice he was given in our clinic. This enabled him to regain confidence in his own intestines and learn to control and take care of his digestive system. His intestinal disorder is in full remission, and for a year he has not had an acute outbreak.

Irritable bowel syndrome (IBS, sometimes referred to as just irritable bowel) is a functional disorder characterized by alterations to the functioning of the digestive system without structural anomalies in the digestive tract. It is one of the most frequently diagnosed gastrointestinal disorders.

The global picture for the prevalence of IBS is far from complete, with no data available for several countries. Published rates are likely to be underestimates because only 25–30 percent of patients with IBS symptoms seek medical attention.

Many people with the symptoms of irritable bowel syndrome simply suffer in silence, frequently because they feel shame in talking about their illness or because they don't consider it sufficiently important. In other cases, they have suffered from it for so long that they don't believe they can live in any other way or get help to improve their condition. They are kept away from the doctor's consulting room by fear, embarrassment, the fact their symptoms are only mild, or the misperception that no effective treatments are available.

What is remarkable is that the available data suggests that the prevalence of IBS is quite similar across many countries, despite substantial lifestyle differences. The prevalence of IBS in Europe and North America (for both children and adults) is estimated to be 10–15 percent, although it is thought to be slightly lower in Sweden. In the Asia–Pacific region the rate is estimated to be 15.9 percent, particularly in countries with developing economies. It is a worrying and obstinate medical problem that takes up a lot of doctors' time.

The clinical and economic importance of irritable bowel syndrome grows ever greater because one of the difficulties for health services is to diagnose the condition with the minimum of tests, given that there are no physiological, biochemical, or visual markers to yield a precise diagnosis. As a result, the final diagnosis can only be based on symptoms; IBS is diagnosed via exclusion of other digestive system diseases or conditions.

Irritable bowel syndrome is an illness that affects above all those with a high level of responsibility and in some studies has been shown to constitute 25–40 percent of diagnoses delivered by doctors specializing in the digestive system. In general, it is the seventh most frequent diagnosis reached by doctors.

Patients with irritable bowel syndrome frequently take days off work, visit the doctor often, and have a diminished quality of life.

IBS is associated with assorted symptoms. It is characterized by various uncomfortable sensations and abdominal pain, diarrhea, and constipation. Sometimes patients experience these symptoms in alternation, as well as an almost continuous sensation of abdominal distension (bloating) produced by gas and intestinal spasms. Another indicator is acute sensitivity to certain foods and stress.

Irritable bowel syndrome is not caused by an infectious agent. However, it has been noticed that in situations of dysbiosis (an imbalance in the intestinal microflora) outbreaks of IBS appear with greater frequency and seriousness (intensity).

Food allergy and leaky gut syndrome are almost always associated with IBS. They can be either the consequences of a chronic digestive inflammation and dysbiosis, related to IBS, or an undiagnosed food allergy, as well as a damaged inner intestinal membrane (which turns out to be leaky), both of which can be the initial causes that provoke the development of IBS. Each clinical case is different. A detailed interview with the patient and a test for food intolerances enables a more precise diagnostic.

A patient can turn out to be hypersensitive to various foods, although it has been observed that the principal foods to which irritable bowel syndrome patients are intolerant are: wheat, yeast, milk, fats, alcohol, coffee, beer, and eggs. Eating a lot of foods containing fiber and wholewheat often makes the situation worse, exacerbating abdominal distension and the pain. This does not mean that a person with IBS cannot eat these foods, only that in the acute phases of the illness it can be beneficial to limit these foods in the diet.

Gas, spasms, and contractions of the intestinal muscles are some of the "tyrannical" symptoms that make patients double up in pain or go rushing to the toilet. Abdominal spasms can become very painful and, in turn, these "knots" block the passage of gas, making the flatulence worse. The irritation and pain culminate in frequent, uncontrollable anal "explosions": attempts by the colon to get rid of its contents.

IBS is often a chronic condition and stays with the patient for years. Sometimes, a visit to the doctor is prompted by light symptoms, but in other cases, it can cause serious upheavals to the patient's daily life.

* * * * * * * *

I greatly admire the literary work of Vladimir Nabokov—not only *Lolita*, his best-known work, but also his short stories, other novels, letters, and university lectures, which shine with rich details and deep analysis of the human soul. His acute sarcasm and his ability with words to describe ordinary events down to the last detail impress me enormously and make me appreciate the simple things in life and notice the little moments of each day.

In his last work, *The Original of Laura* (which was recovered after his death and published in 2009), Nabokov gives a perfect description of IBS—which also reminds us that intestinal neurosis frequently coincides with the low self-esteem of the sufferer: "I loathe my belly, that trunkful of bowels, which I have to carry around, and everything connected with it—the wrong food, heartburn, constipation's leaden load, or else indigestion with a first instalment of hot filth pouring out of me in a public toilet three minutes before a punctual engagement."

Stress, anxiety, and depression can make symptoms worse and provoke fresh acute outbreaks. Irritable bowel syndrome is closely linked to the psychoemotional state of the person, to the point that it could be considered more a psychological than digestive disorder. There are studies that show the development of IBS in people with traumatic childhoods involving abuse and episodes of violence.

To understand the functional upheavals of the colon we have to return to the subject of our second brain.

It has been established that the enteric neurons (the cells of the digestive nervous system, or the neurons of the second brain) release various neurotransmitters, the most important being acetylcholine, norepinephrine, nitric oxide, vasoactive intestinal peptide, and serotonin.

Seretonin is produced by the enterochromaffin cells in the gastric epithelium. These cells are activated by pressure stimuli such as, for example, those caused by the passage of a bolus through the digestive tube. The secreted serotonin stimulates the nerves that regulate the peristaltic reflex.

It has been shown that 90 percent of the body's serotonin, the neurotransmitter that influences mood and creates a sensation of calm and well-being, is produced by the enteric brain, which can also experience its own type of neurosis. Scientists consider that the enteric nervous system (our second brain) can remember certain emotions and suffer from stress. The neurons in your intestines not only control digestion; they also produce psychoactive substances that influence mood and synthesizing benzodiazepines, which have a tranquilizing effect.

Everything indicates that irritable bowel syndrome originates in the intestinal brain, or at least that it is involved in some fundamental way. Intestinal symptoms illuminate the personality and psychic conflicts. Insecurity, fear, anger, control, and other similar feelings lead to retention, and consequently constipation, intestinal ulcers, or a spastic colon.

In the intestines, where internal and external realities meet, aspects of our personality can be stored and it can be scary to unleash them.

· · · · · · · · ·

N., an emotionally scarred and unhappy young woman, couldn't see anything in a positive light, nor any way out of her problems. She suffered from tremendous bloating, abdominal pains, and constipation, alternating with periods of diarrhea. Her digestive system had to work hard, and she couldn't tolerate some foods. All this is compatible with an irritable bowel. After each fight or frustrating confrontation with her partner, her neurotic intestine almost disabled her, beginning with intestinal spasms and digestive blocks.

She had to make a big effort to learn to look after herself and restore her digestive functions. It has been a long journey with many detours, but she has achieved her goal. In N.'s case it was especially important to arrange a program of psychological work and sessions of guided visualization to enable her to reconnect with her inner self, and to recognize her own personality and needs. It is as if she has at last learned to listen to her gut, her second brain. Having recovered her strength and confidence, she is full of light and positivity and complies with all the treatments of detoxification and nutrition that she is given. Her digestive system is still fragile and sensitive, but it has recovered and her colon is now back under control.

Emotions play a fundamental role in enteric upsets. Almost all patients with irritable bowel syndrome have mental and emotional problems, such as anxiety, fatigue, aggression, and disturbed sleep. One theory suggests that those who suffer with their digestive nervous system do so because they developed such problems in childhood as a means of coping with stressful situations. As children they learned to transform their problems into actual physical symptoms, thereby taking the spotlight off more deep-seated emotional difficulties.

Diarrhea, for example, can be the result of fear, which multiplies the stimuli affecting the circuits that produce serotonin.

· · · · · · · ·

A patient of mine with irritable bowel syndrome told me of an outbreak of acute diarrhea that occurred because she was going through a divorce.

Another, a young man, experiences a painful, frothy discharge of his gut every Sunday after having lunch with his mother. Traumatic memories of his infancy are recorded in his two brains, and his relationship with his mother causes him much pain and anger.

In a detailed interview, a patient with IBS will often recover distant memories of some difficult and repeated emotional situation where his only means of escape was abdominal pain. Intestinal upsets, therefore, can reveal a difficulty in confronting the obstacles of life. To help such patients is a great challenge.

On that note, let's now return to the subject of the two human brains, and the different ways they influence each other and alternate functions.

We have already seen that the intestinal consequences of strong emotions are neither esoteric nor merely theoretical: for the majority of people they are real problems of everyday life. The brain is an obvious author of intestinal pain. Anxiety, a fight using angry words, an emotional conflict, disappointment—any of these may be accompanied by diarrhea or intestinal cramps. Some people are so used to the music of their intestines that if they didn't have them they wouldn't know when they were anxious or stressed.

The gut brain, however, can cause intestinal dysfunction by itself, without the participation or influence of the higher brain. The aches and pains in the abdomen that a patient describes can be real, unleashed by physical or chemical abnormalities in the intestines, with consequential changes to the patient's mood or personality. In Argentina, people use an interesting word to describe this bridge between the physical and emotional: *entripado* — a word that can be used to describe strong stomach pains, extreme anger, or emotional exhaustion.

There is a scientific explanation as to why the stomach "closes up" in a stressful situation or seems to be filled with butterflies when you are in love: changes in the second brain, the ENS. When we talk about "irritable" bowel, we mean that the nerve endings in the walls of the intestines are unusually sensitive, that the nerves that control the musculature of the intestines are unusually hyperactive, and that the neurons in the ENS are producing excessive quantities of neurotransmitters to manage this.

As a result of this irritability, the gut responds in an exaggerated fashion to an event that may be totally normal, such as the transit of certain foods, gas, or liquids through it, by causing inappropriate muscular activity, which can momentarily interrupt the intestinal flow or lead to the overwhelming necessity to expel material from the intestine at an inconvenient moment. Abdominal distension is the most conspicuous symptom, and can become obvious in the person affected by IBS. It is never constant, and it can appear and reappear within a short period. It typically gets worse during the day but rarely at night. It is said to be an illness that lets you sleep.

IBS also gets worse and causes fresh outbreaks of symptoms in situations of tiredness, exhaustion, and lack of sleep. It may also react to spicy food, alcohol, and certain medications. For example, in the American comedy film *Along Came Polly*, we break up laughing when we see the protagonist, played by Ben Stiller, suffer an attack of IBS after a meal of ethnic food. The poor man ends up in a ridiculous and shameful situation, destroying the bathroom of his girlfriend (Jennifer Aniston). In his case, the IBS appears suddenly for two reasons: the nervousness of the young man possibly embarking on a romantic relationship, combined with the effects of the spicy food.

Anyone who suffers from IBS won't find this funny; scenarios like this really do happen. For example, on starting a new relationship they set out to make an impression in bed but end their night on the toilet. The same can happen in the workplace when faced with having to do a presentation, meet with the boss, or appear in front of a tribunal. It is highly frustrating to know that your intestinal brain can let you down at the most critical moment, at the culmination of some important transaction. In the above-mentioned film, the same subject is used to make us laugh at the character played by Philip Seymour Hoffman (the friend of the main character) who soils himself at an art exhibition, sighing that he only thought he was letting out a fart. You never know…

In cases of frequent episodes of diarrhea, the acidic feces irritate the anus, provoking stinging, inflammation, and pain in the rectal area. This can lead to temporary incontinence or the inability to distinguish between gas and liquid. It is a significant disorder that is difficult to treat and control. Those who suffer from it don't usually talk about it or ask for help—until, that is, it leads to a fissure or bleeding hemorrhoids (piles).

For many years, people with chronic abdominal pain were told that it was imaginary or emotional. Patients who appear in surgeries with problems that can't be solved or clearly diagnosed are often classified as mentally instable. In the daily practice of medicine, unfortunately, many doctors conclude that patients with functional disorders of the intestines, including IBS, are merely worried and preoccupied with their gut, and that their complaints are minor and their pain minimal. How can we know that the pain described by our patients is minimal? When we do not find visual evidence to confirm what our patients are telling us, we classify these afflictions as psychogenic in origin, and we don't offer any help.

If, instead, the complaint is about another organ, such as the heart, we doctors believe what we are told; we don't doubt the patient for a moment when he describes his pain. There is no reason to treat the digestive system in a different way from the cardiovascular system. Agreed?

## Alternative Treatments

From a holistic point of view, the treatment of an irritable intestine begins with a localized therapy: hydrotherapy of the colon (colonic cleansing). Its objectives are to:

- Detoxify and clean the intestinal walls of old residues and gas that have accumulated, loosening deposits that have hardened and concentrated there over many years and that irritate the mucosa;
- Decongest the large intestine, to improve transit;
- Activate the process of regeneration of the mucosa lining of the intestines;
- Balance the ecology and the pH of the intestines;
- Relax spasms and muscular contractions, balancing the motility of the intestines; and
- Reduce irritation and local hypersensitivity in the intestine.

Localized treatment helps the intestinal mucosa heal itself and allows irritation to subside. It is a quick and efficient way to influence an intestinal environment that has become too aggressive, acidic, and out of ecological balance.

Compare this to what happens with irritation we experience on the outside of our body. When we have an area of skin that has become irritated or sensitive due, perhaps, to dermatitis or a light sunburn, we automatically try to cover it so that it is not exposed to any further irritation. We likely use a soothing cream and try to keep it dry, if we can. This is logical, because if this area of skin gets moist or dirty recovery will slow down, and it will take longer to return to its healthy state and fulfil its functions. It's the same inside the body. If we take care of an exaggerated local sensitivity—an acute irritation of the intestines—it will clear up more quickly.

In colonic hydrotherapy, we use purified, distilled water that may be enriched with ozone and mixed with infusions of medicinal plants and individualized preparations of *probiotics* ("friendly" bacteria that are beneficial to intestinal microflora—the colon needs these to nourish itself and boost the immune system).

Without doubt, colonic hydrotherapy brings tremendous relief to people who suffer from IBS and results in immediate and clear improvement in the state of the intestines. To achieve a prolonged remission, however, it is essential that the patient has full confidence in the process and is willing to follow therapeutic and nutritional instructions after their treatment.

Colonic hydrotherapy treatment produces immediate results. The patient notices a sense of relief and an impressive diminution of symptoms. Nevertheless, the duration of this curative effect depends on the behavior and the attitude of the patient afterwards. The diet and food supplements detailed below are essential in order to achieve a long term remission.

During the colonic cleansing, the intestinal lumen (the space enclosed by the intestinal walls) is cleared, the muscles relax, and this, in turn, helps to eliminate the gas and the toxic residues "trapped" in the digestive tract. Little by little, the water flowing through the colon loosens and eliminates old and encrusted fecal and bilious materials that are generally stuck to the intestinal walls and that keep the intestines in a state of irritation and inflammation. Colonic irrigation helps to get rid of any old and dead cells and compressed mucus produced by the interaction between the mucosa and bacteria. These substances are normal and present in small quantities in a healthy colon, but where there is localized and persistent inflammation they accumulate in the intestinal tract in alarming quantities, "covering" the lumen and preventing the intestinal epithelium from being adequately nourished.

Little by little, under the gentle but insistent pressure of the water, the overgrown colonies of pathological bacterial growths—fungi; parasites; fecal, bilious, and other stones; and crystals of various salts and minerals—flush out of the colon through the tubes of the hydrotherapy machine.

Patients sometimes ask me why we clean the intestines with water, when they are suffering from diarrhea? And, if only a malodorous liquid comes out, is the intestine clean? We must return to the comparison with damaged skin to answer this—the cut or external wound that we imagined as inflamed and oozing pus. A health practitioner (or you yourself) will clean the area well with a curative solution, dry it, apply a disinfectant or calmative ointment, and keep it covered. We treat the intestines in a similar manner: cleaning the irritated area, hydrating it, relaxing it, and calming it down while we apply a remedy.

People with an irritable colon frequently find that they experience alternating episodes of diarrhea and constipation. They rely on these "pauses" to provide rest and (relative) peace in their gut, but this slowing down of intestinal transit isn't a good sign, either. After suffering bouts of diarrhea, the colon is moist but tired, its mucosa stretched and the bacteria living there confused and dizzy. This is a good moment to apply a strict diet, almost a fast. To fill the inflamed intestine with new waste matter and leave it like this for several days would mean inducing new outbreaks or episodes and more protests.

## Dietary Advice for IBS

If for some reason you cannot have a colonic hydrotherapy treatment, I recommend you at least observe a special diet and take nutritional supplements right after episodes of diarrhea. Relaxation and breathing exercises and abdominal massage are also of great help. This should take just 15–20 minutes a day, but your gut will thank you. The diet recommended for an irritable colon is as follows:

### AVOID

- Products made with wheat flour (bread, pasta, wheat cereals, breaded products) but you can eat other cereals and/or gluten-free products
- Milk (except in dairy products mentioned below)
- Sugar, sweets, and chocolate
- Soft drinks, beer, and alcohol, in general
- Raw vegetables (except when juiced or puréed), including tomatoes, peppers, and aubergines
- Pulses (legumes)
- Oranges
- Wholewheat products with a lot of fiber, bran, or seeds. Brown rice (but you can eat white rice).
- Dried fruits and nuts (except nut butters)
- Commercial sauces and condiments
- Strongly flavored or fatty processed meat products, such as sausages, smoked ham, etc.
- Fried foods
- Mature and semi-mature cheeses.

## EAT

- Lean meats and fish roasted or baked in the oven or grilled (accompanied by white rice and cooked or steamed vegetables)
- Grilled, boiled, steamed, or roasted vegetables (best in the form of creams and purées)
- Fermented (cultured) dairy products, such as plain yogurt, kefir, fresh cheeses, and curds
- White rice
- Oats (porridge, or oatmeal, is a good option for breakfast or dinner)
- No more than two slices of rye, spelt, gluten-free, or potato bread for breakfast (substitute rice or corn cakes)
- Peeled fruit including apples, pears, peaches, apricots, melon and watermelon, blackberries and raspberries, bananas, and lemons. Check your sensitivity in case of grapefruits, mandarins, and strawberries. Neither plums nor grapes are recommended.
- Honey
- For snacks and dessert, oats, rice pudding, natural low-fat yogurt, and fruit are recommended.

## REMEMBER

- Eat slowly and chew well.
- Drink at least 2 liters of filtered water daily, along with lots of herbal tea.
- Eat small, balanced meals every four hours, and don't overeat. Give your digestive system an opportunity to recover after the earthquake it has gone through.
- Take high-quality probiotics. These are natural supplements that contain therapeutic levels of friendly bacteria to balance your intestinal microflora.
- Include a source of soluble fiber (the type that forms a gel in water and soothes the gut), such as psyllium, inulin, or flaxseed.

In order to see a difference I urge you to follow the above diet, supplements, and other therapeutic advice for at least a month. If that is not possible, try to at least stick to the protocol for five days after an IBS episode. Why five days? Because this is the minimum time needed for the relining of the digestive tract; it is thought that within this period the body has time to grow new cells and restore the mucosa.

Have you ever watched how animals (pets, for example) overcome their digestive problems and illnesses? It is very curious. They act on an instinctive level, perceiving the signals of their intestinal brains. Normally when cats and dogs fall ill, they fast, drink a lot of water, and lie down and sleep a lot, taking all the time and space they need to cure themselves. Cats look for fresh grass to eat, and sometimes they make themselves vomit, enabling them to clean their insides. Dogs suddenly show an interest in vegetables.

Human beings are equally intuitive, and we have a great potential for internal self-cure. Children in their first years of life are somewhat similar in their behavior to animals until they become completely conditioned by adults and their social environment.

· · · · · · · · ·

A desperate mother brought her 9-year-old son to my consulting room. This child had an expression of suffering on his face, and he listened and passed opinions on his painful gut as if he were an adult. The boy had had chronic constipation since birth, along with bloating (an excess of gas in the intestine and abdominal swelling) and colic, and he bled when he expelled the hard plugs of feces that formed. He was used to being attended to by the medical emergency services. Each night, his mother gave him a laxative or inserted a rectal suppository. He was well informed about the limits of his diet: he had to eat vegetables and fiber essentially and it made him very sad not to be able to eat rich and exciting food like his "healthy" friends.

The inflammation in the boy's digestive system reached its limits, and his intestines began to make their condition known through acute episodes of diarrhea and anal incontinence. He couldn't control his sphincter, and he never knew whether gas or feces would come out. At nine years old he was soiling himself, and his schoolmates—alerted by the smell—made cruel jokes at his expense. The psychological consequences of his condition now dominated his life. The child told me, "Now I have liquid farts, and I don't know what to do." It brought a lump to my throat to listen to such a fragile young child suffering so much.

I would love there to be training courses on basic digestive health and nutrition for children and parents. This would prevent many problems of both physical and emotional health and improve the quality of life for new generations.

This child had symptoms compatible with an irritable bowel, but in his case we couldn't rule out some other condition: malabsorption, serious food intolerances, an infection, or another pathology. It was essential to carry out in-depth medical tests. At the same time, it was necessary to establish some order in this little digestive system, starting with a diet that totally excluded all dairy and wheat derivatives—I know this was not easy for a child of his age—and very selective treatment with various probiotics and enzyme products.

The fact that the child had been diagnosed with bronchial asthma and had problems of attention suggested that he had very probably developed a high level of intestinal permeability (leaky gut syndrome) and that he suffered from multiple food intolerances. In order to help this mother and child we had to devise a scheme of work adapted to their needs.

Let me repeat that people who suffer from IBS should look at this condition in a focused, integrated, holistic way, treating all the physical and psychological aspects of the illness together.

# Natural Remedies

### Magnesium

Taken as a dietary supplement or in special mineral waters, magnesium improves intestinal transit, stimulating the muscles of the digestive tube and obliging it to make gentle cyclical movements so that it moves the remains of food in the right direction. Magnesium teaches the digestive system to organize its motility without provoking additional irritation to the mucosa. It also alkalizes the body and has an "antistress" effect at the level of the enteric nervous system. In addition, this mineral activates the function of the gallbladder and the bile ducts.

You have to be careful with the dose of magnesium and the choice of its chemical form, because in too high doses and in more active forms (such as magnesium sulfate), it can accelerate the intestinal rhythm too much and provoke soft stools. However, in the form of magnesium carbonate or a dietary mineral, magnesium can help control the "mood swings" of your gut. I recommend that you always consult a health professional to make sure that the form of magnesium used is the right one for you and that you take the correct dose.

### Ground Psyllium Seed Husks

Psyllium (*Plantago ovato*) is a plant that dilutes well in water to form a gel that lubricates the digestive tract. As it passes through, it protects the intestinal walls, hydrating and gently stimulating the intestinal muscles. In addition, this fiber serves as a good source of nutrition for the intestinal microflora and impedes the absorption of toxins. In cases of diarrhea, psyllium helps to "switch off" the irritation and its fiber content encourages well-formed feces. In cases of constipation, it works as a laxative of mass: it fills the intestinal space and, by increasing its volume, applies a gentle pressure on the intestine from the lumen; this stimulates the muscles of the walls and provokes "waves" that increase the motility. Some patients, however, have such serious intestinal problems that psyllium doesn't have any positive effect on them and can increase the sensation of bloating.

## Flaxseeds

Another way to lubricate and reduce inflammation in the intestines is to take flaxseeds, either whole or ground, previously soaked in water. Flax releases mucilage that has a healing and calming effect on the mucosa. Being a water-soluble fiber with nutritive properties, it also helps regularize intestinal transit time.

## Aloe Vera

There are many myths around the famous aloe vera plant. Personally, I have a lot of respect for this natural remedy, and I always recommend using it in the form of the living plant or as a fresh preparation made by hand. The list of magical properties of aloe vera is endless, and the history of its use goes back thousands of years. The flesh of aloe vera has anti-inflammatory properties; it calms and heals the digestive system; it helps restore the pH balance; it improves the intestinal microflora; and it cures erosion and ulceration. It is excellent in cases of allergies and food intolerances.

All of the above healing properties correspond *only* to the soft inner part of the leaves of aloe vera. It is very important to remember to use only the inside of fresh leaves (the transparent, gelatinous pulp that is evident when you cut open the plant). You need to extract this internal substance and discard the dense, dark green skin of the leaves. The pulp of aloe vera can be mashed up or mixed with honey, wine, water, or taken in concentrated form—but no more than a tablespoonful of the fresh preparation before each main meal. It can also be used in salads and in various juices.

The skin of aloe vera contains bitter compounds that act as an irritant laxative. Because of this herbalists frequently recommend aloe vera for constipation. It is not good to use it to treat an irritable colon and certainly not for a prolonged period. I repeat: only the inner part—not the skin—is calmative, curative, and anti-inflammatory. When you buy an aloe vera preparation make sure that it doesn't have traces of skin in it. A much better and healthier idea is to keep your own plant at home, given that it is not demanding and grows well. That way, you can use its leaves when the need arises.

## Other Medicinal Plants

In cases of symptoms compatible with acute intestinal neurosis, you can use the following plants to good effect: valerian, passionflower, California poppy, hops, and St. John's wort.

## Mint Tea

In some patients, infusions of mint have a significant antispasmodic effect. Peppermint oil in enteric capsules has been shown to be effective in more than 16 controlled clinical studies. Some researchers now consider it as a medicine of first resort for IBS when not accompanied by serious diarrhea or constipation.

Note: When I make comments about the use of natural remedies, I am always referring to a course of treatment lasting several months at least. This is the time necessary to have a good therapeutic effect, because medicinal plants are more gentle in their action in comparison with drugs and take time to reach curative levels in the body. Taking alternative and complementary medications is a ritual and a daily reconnection with nature; you have to trust the process, be disciplined with the dosage, and be patient.

## Probiotics and Prebiotics

Probiotics are living bacteria that are administered in capsules or in powder, or which are found incorporated in yogurt or kefir. They help restore the equilibrium of the intestinal flora and have positive effects on the immune system. It is important to get the correct dosage of each preparation before it is introduced into the intestines. You also need to insure that these preparations contain living organisms in a pure form without additives, and that they are in the appropriate formulations able to survive the journey to the colon. There are a lot of products available on the market, and I strongly recommend seeking professional advice on which is best. It is better to use these preparations without mixing different strains, alternating lactobacillus, bifidus, and acidophilus (the three most typical types of probiotic).

In my consulting room, I have noticed that some patients who take remedies for their intestinal microflora that are based on various yeasts (such as brewer's) experience an increase in flatulence. This is due to the presence of food intolerances or candidiasis (overgrowth of yeast in the body). When you start to take a new dietary supplement, you have to monitor the response of your digestive system with great attention.

Prebiotics are a combination of different types of fiber that serve as nutrients for "good" bacteria and for the intestinal epithelium. The most common of them is inulin, which can be taken, for example, in powdered form, as tablets, or in plum juice.

The daily consumption of various cocktails of juices and vegetables ensures an adequate supplement of prebiotics (the liquidized form liberates more of the essential fiber and pectin).

## Hypnotherapy

Hypnotherapy has long been recognized as a valuable treatment for IBS, and in the UK, specialized hypnotherapy departments have been operating as part of the National Health Service (NHS) since 2002. Around 80 percent of patients show a sustained improvement in their symptoms after several sessions of hypnotherapy. Hypnotherapy has also been shown to alleviates symptoms outside the colon, improving patient quality of life and helping IBS sufferers get back to work.

A very common notion is that hypnotherapy involves the subject being put to sleep—or half to sleep—and then being given suggestions by the therapist to do odd things, such as levitate. Prejudices and ignorance of hypnotherapy can lead to the false belief that someone can temporarily dominate your consciousness, navigating your relaxed mind. This is not true. Therapeutic hypnosis involves relaxation but in a fully conscious state. In my experience, a few sessions of Eriksonian hypnosis, together with exercises of guided visualization, produces a notable improvement in patients suffering from functional digestive upsets that are rooted in certain psychological states.

Another technique that has been demonstrated to be effective is the "shamanic journey." This is a process of visualization induced by the regular beating of a drum (either in person or via a recording). Because of their particular frequency, the drum enables the brain to go into a relaxed state and visualize with greater clarity, generating images of the possible causes of the problem as well as the possible solutions. Of course, this has to be under the personal supervision of a therapist, who helps the patient to understand the messages of his brain. They are called shamanic journeys because they originate in the ancient wisdom of shamans from diverse cultures around the world. Dr. Michael Hartner, an anthropologist specializing in shamanic cultures and traditions, has studied the process in various ancient societies and has adapted it for the urban lifestyle of the West, so that we can reap the benefits of these techniques in our daily life. Psychological work in small groups, and sessions of couple or family therapy, can also be a great help in stabilizing a digestive neurosis.

## Yoga

Some yoga movements and postures appear to be of benefit to patients with IBS. Controlled clinical studies of young and adult patients with irritable bowel syndrome who were asked to practise 12 asanas (yoga postures) for two months have demonstrated that this technique of relaxation is more effective than the drug loperamide in the control of diarrhea. The postures employed, in combination with appropriate breathing techniques, help relax the abdominal muscles, expel gas, and improve peristalsis.

The "gut," our innards, is, in my understanding, the visceral behavior of our consciousness. Sometimes we feel an emotion in our guts before we are able to identify it and put it into words. On many occasions our gut urges us on, making us act, or express that which is about to become conscious and which intimidates us or frightens us (movements of the intestines, explosions, protests, discharges…); they speak the truth when we insist on denying it.

Dr. Irina guides us in a passionate, creative, and informed way; she shows us how to unravel the secrets of this subsystem of our bodies.

In spite of my medical training, until I had a consultation with Irina, I had not found better advice to alleviate the various food intolerances and digestive upsets that I have suffered from since childhood than the well-intentioned words grownups would tell me, paraphrasing the advice of Don Quixote to Sancho Panza: "Eat little and dine even less; the health of the whole body is forged in the workshop of the stomach." Later he adds: "Drink moderately; bear in mind that wine doesn't keep secrets or keep its word," and, "Remember, Sancho, not to eat noisily, and don't burp in front of people…"

Now we have a valuable and practical alternative. This book is an intelligent, informed document that integrates modern advances in the science of health with nutrition at a time when, more than ever, we are conscious of the need to take care of our diet and our bodies, in order to reach higher levels of health and well-being.

Dr. Irina is an excellent, dedicated, and intuitive practitioner who has the rare gift of drawing together knowledge from the most diverse disciplines, making her work an art.

— *ANA MARIA RUIZ SANCHO*, MD, PSYCHIATRIST, PSYCHOTHERAPIST, CONSULTANT IN GROUP AND ORGANIZATIONAL DYNAMICS. FOUNDER AND DIRECTOR OF VOCACCION.

4

# A Social Taboo

We do not know at exactly which moment in history our gut—the functioning of the intestines, in particular—came to be thought of as so tremendously unwholesome and shameful; a matter not worthy of our attention and certainly not to be talked about in society.

Our digestive functions are very intimate and not easy for us to understand. Digestion takes its own course according to multiple internal programs, and all that we want is for it not to cause us any trouble or leave us with disagreeable memories. Curiously, it is easier and more acceptable for us to talk about sex, but we wouldn't think of discussing or gossiping about our digestion and defecation in the same way.

As a rule, most of us are conditioned by family and society; we accord great importance to the judgments and opinions of others and allow them to overrule our nature. Without social recognition, we wouldn't be sure of our own identities. Our digestive behavior is similarly subject to social, educational, and family influences.

· · · · · · · ·

One of my patients confessed to me that he had been a nervous, hyperactive child, and so as not to lose play time he had suppressed the need to defecate until he soiled himself or until he had strong colic pains (a consequence of the gas produced by retaining his feces). This made him the subject of jokes by his companions. Recorded in his infant memory is the notion that to defecate is bad and shameful, that to move one's bowels is annoying and disagreeable. When he grew up he developed chronic constipation, with its toxic overload, and on more than one occasion he ended up in the hospital emergency room.

His own processes of digestion and excretion caused him to react with negativity and repugnance; because of this, he ignored them and seriously failed to take care of himself. It took him an enormous effort to recover his natural reflexes and learn to respect his digestive system.

Another patient, as an adolescent, grew used to retaining his gas and feces because of a violent family atmosphere (fear of the authority of his father and punishments). He suffered severe abdominal pains and had to make frequent trips to the ER. He had suffered a childhood psychological trauma and was somatizing it in his intestines.

Now, as a young man, he has chronic problems, both digestive and psychological, and needs continual medication.

Let's get back to history.

The practice of purges, diets, and fasts, and the use of medicinal plants as aids to
digestive health, has a history going back thousands of years.

The cult of intestinal hygiene was an important part of the life of the pharaohs of
ancient Egypt. Egyptian priests observed how the sacred bird, the ibis, introduced its
beak into its anus to blow water up it and thus clean its intestines. This practice was
adopted by the pharaohs.

The guardian of the pharaoh's anus was a prestigious position. The work of the
office holder consisted in blowing water through a golden tube in order to clean the
noble anus after a large meal.

In ancient China, to have a bloated and dirty gut was deemed to be bad-mannered
and meant that dark, negative energy had accumulated inside; if it was unable to flow
out, it caused internal damage. This continues to be the most important principle of
traditional Chinese medicine.

In India, the treatments of Ayurvedic medicine are concentrated on cleaning the
body and its energy; these are considered the root of health and balance.

An apocryphal book in the Bible explains how to clean the body to facilitate spiritual purity by means of an enema using a gourd. Once this had been hollowed out,
it is ready for use as a recipient. It had to be placed in a bush, filled with water, and
connected to the intestines by means of a hollow stalk, so that the water could be
introduced.

Earlier ages were less prudish than we are about bodily functions. In ancient
Rome, philosophical and rhetorical meetings took place in public toilets. Their citi-
zens knew that a good digestion favored clear thoughts and fostered intelligence and
a good mood. There are old engravings that show benches of stone or clay, hollow
inside, arranged in a square. Each bench had several holes to sit on. It was probably
one of the first prototypes for a public toilet. Bearded philosophers would sit there,
in front of each other, showing respect for each other's physiological needs while they
discussed poetry, mathematics, and astronomy.

Even in those days, they instinctively knew about intestinal hygiene and there was
nothing shameful or prohibited about the guts.

In Europe during the Middle Ages, all aspects of digestion were considered part
of life. To defecate and let out gas—without moving out of the way—was not considered something bad but rather the expression of human nature. Because of a lack
of hygiene, human waste was not cleaned up. As a consequence, throughout history,

violent epidemics have rampaged through the population, killing thousands of people within months.

Around this time, doctors and faith healers in Europe began to advocate cleanliness, a minimal digestive hygiene and the use of natural disinfectants.

The medieval church took note of the need to change practices of hygiene. It began to separate sick people in monastery and convent infirmaries, use aromatic incense during mass, and to proclaim cleanliness as desirable to God. The first public baths appeared, and with them new social norms.

In later ages, blue-blooded members of the nobility sought to separate themselves from the common people by taking care of themselves. Fragrances were used, and clean baths and special underwear were favored. However, information about digestion was not widely diffused, even among the aristocracy.

In France, the residences of Versailles and Fontainebleau are renowned for their magnificent and luxurious architecture. The beauty of their halls and salons impresses the visitor, but interestingly there are no bathrooms, nor any trace of a toilet. (The first simple bathroom and toilet, of military design, appeared later, in the time of Napoleon.) Digestive rituals were carried out with complete naturalness, using porcelain jars from the palace as chamber pots in the salons themselves. Servants would empty the contents of these receptacles in the gardens, not far away.

Everything was gossiped about and discussed by the court. Nothing was out of bounds nor considered shameful—from the color of the kings chronic diarrhea to the color of the dresses of the season. Louis XIV didn't like to wash, so throughout his life servants washed him with moist aromatic towels. As a result, this practice was observed by many faithful courtiers, too.

The Sun King had digestive problems that seem to have been related to overeating. The solution adopted was copied from ancient Egypt: to carry out enemas "in regal style," using gold tubes and rose and lavender water. It is documented that during his lifetime, Louis XIV received more than 2,000 enemas to keep him in good shape. Courtiers discussed the king's enemas and, of course, all of them emulated him. The Sun King died at the age of 77, having been king for 72 years. For the standards of his time, he had a long, healthy life, and his mind was lucid until the end.

With the development of medicine and sanitation, we were able to start to distance ourselves from monitoring our gut health. After the discovery of antibiotics, we decided that we no longer needed enemas as we now had magic pills available to deal with all of our ills. Because of strong and complex social pressures, we have come to see our own entrails as dirty and smelly—a reminder that we, too, are animals. To expel air through the entrance or exit of the digestive system is impolite, and to talk about digestion and defecation is considered bad taste.

We have forgotten that being in touch with our natural body need not be incompatible with living in modern society, but our children remind us. We teach children how and where to carry out their digestive functions. When a child accidentally soils himself or farts as a joke, teachers with good manners say, "That's not good. You can't do that!" We tell children what is prohibited but don't emphasise what is commendable. In general, we don't bother, or consider it essential, to explain to children that it is very good and important to go to the toilet every day, and that feces and gas have to come out; that these things are a part of life; that they are natural and necessary; and that they enable us to grow and to be clean and healthy.

It would be wonderful if we could start to educate children to attend to their needs naturally, each morning, alone in the toilet, making it clear that this is not ugly but simply something personal and intimate that doesn't need to be shared. Children are wonderful, they get the message quickly, and they do it very well.

*In these few lines I would like to express my gratitude to Irina, a great friend and magnificent doctor. Thanks to her, I have learned to listen to my body and to understand the way in which food and the digestive process is linked to the emotions. To know how to eat is not only a pleasure, it also serves to make us aware that the object of alimentation is to generate healthy energy and that we can feel strong and full of vitality. For this reason, we have to give up those foods that cost us more energy to digest than we get back from them and that only serve to poison us, leaving us physically and psychologically exhausted.*

*The first time that I had a consultation with Irina, my only obsession was my problem of being overweight. To solve this has been a complicated process, because it coincided with various endocrinal and emotional problems. To find a solution has not been an easy task. After four years, thanks to Irina, I have learned to control my metabolic problems through an adequate diet and three or four hours of moderate exercise each week. I have discovered that cleaning the colon can lead to a physical balance that transcends the mental in a spectacular way, which results in a considerable boost to well-being and beauty. I have learned to listen to my emotions, feelings, and the way they are linked to food. It is impossible to be healthy if we don't look after our insides. To understand all that we are told, the digestive process, the adequate combination of foods, the importance of the intestine and its care, the food that suits us, and how to influence our psyches… is a passionate quest, which gets you hooked. I urge you to read this book and to enjoy the holistic experience of putting it into practice.*

— **TERESA BUEYES HERNANDEZ**, *LAWYER*

# 5

# The Stomach

*"My stomach is making noises."*
*"I have stomachache."*
*"My stomach is empty."*
*"I have stomach problems."*
*"I have a delicate stomach."*
*"Why is my stomach bloated, and why does it produce gas?"*
*"My stomach is really swollen."*
*"I have a knot in my stomach."*
*"I have an upset/unsettled/dodgy stomach."*
*"I have stomach cramps."*
*"I have a pain in the pit of my stomach."*
*"My stomach is swollen like a balloon."*

For many people, the "stomach" means anything below the chest, which leads them to make remarks such as those above. One person is convinced that he has a "stomach of iron" or "like a shark"; another says his stomach is "distended," "closed," "hard," "heavy," or "tight."

These are all common complaints, and they can refer to any problem of the digestive system, not necessarily anything to do with the stomach itself. The job of a doctor is to find out where the breakdown actually is and to determine its causes.

For example, in the majority of cases of intestinal disorder or gallbladder problems, people blame the stomach and believe that all problems are located there, so they must have a slow digestion. But gas and constipation in the intestines can cause inflammation that pushes the stomach upward, and even though the poor organ has nothing to do with the swelling, this pressure can "speak to us," through a sensation of heartburn (and that one originates in the stomach, indeed).

Indeed, it is difficult to distinguish where exactly things inside happen inside us, and because of this we end up attributing everything to the stomach. This happens not out of ignorance but because of history.

## A Short History

For many centuries, the stomach was considered to be the first, and most important, part of the gut. It "talked" to us, using the language of hunger—hunger being an ever-present danger in centuries past, with the power to take away life. To fill the stomach with food meant everything: strength, the power to work, and to avoid becoming "a mere animal motivated by hunger."

The word stomach derives from the Latin *stomachus,* which in turn comes from the Greek *stomachos*, which has as its root *stoma*, meaning "mouth."

Initially, medieval doctors believed the stomach was able "to think"—that it was an active nucleus. Galen of Pergamon (AD 130–200 or 216), the Greek physician whose thinking dominated European medicine for over a thousand years, classed the stomach as a sentient being that could feel its own emptiness and generate the sensation of hunger. In his treatise, *Of the Natural Faculties,* Galen writes: "Nature has conceded to the stomach, and in particular the parts nearest the mouth, the capacity to feel the lack of food. This wakes an animal hunger and initiates the search for food. It is, as well, a warehouse of nutrients."

The doctor and philosopher Avicenna (c. AD 980–1037) recognized the importance of nutrition and the vulnerability of the stomach in illness and gave abundant advice on diet and digestion, writing principally on the stomach and the intestines in relation to these two factors. He observed that "mental excitement and the emotions and vigorous physical exercise make digestion difficult."

The scholar Master Nicholas wrote poetically in the 12th century that "the stomach has below it the liver, just as a fire has beneath it a cauldron: the stomach is like a cooking pot, the gallbladder is the cook, and the liver its fire."

Later, during the Renaissance, doctors presented the complex theory of a stomach as a cold, dry organ that acted as one of the principal organs of the body. The Renaissance artist and anatomist Leonardo da Vinci believed that the digestive system was the principal aid to our respiration.

From all this, we can see that stomach has historically been an "organ-cum-symbol," a way of conceptualizing bad digestion in general, and also our emotional ills.

## Anatomical and Physiological Virtues

The stomach is shaped like a letter "J." It is a dilated section of the alimentary tract, with the muscular "fist" of the esophageal sphincter above it and the pyloric sphincter below it, another "fist," or valve, that regulates the exit of partially processed foods into the small intestine.

The stomach is covered by a mucosa of special epithelial cells under which is a layer of connective tissue. Both layers are strong dense materials that possess a vital quality: they are able to protect themselves from the stomach's own acidity. Below these, there are muscular layers covered with a serous membrane.

An adult stomach is capable of receiving and containing 1–3.5 liters (1.5–6 pints) of foods and liquids and producing 3 liters (5 pints) of gastric juices every 24 hours. Digestion and the absorption of some compounds in our food is carried out in the stomach. During this process, the bolus of the food eaten is converted into *chyme* (a semifluid mush).

The stomach is much more than a pot that is used to prepare an internal "broth" and transport it to the next stretch of the digestive tract. It is lined with a network of intelligent cells that, from the moment we smell food, begin to prepare precise quantities of acids, *enzymes* (protein complexes that produce specific chemical changes in other substances and catalyze chemical reactions without themselves changing), and *hormones,* and to program muscular functions. The stomach secretes water, *electrolytes* (substances that contain free ions), enzymes, and *glycoproteins* (proteins joined to carbohydrates), which intervene in a whole series of physiological processes. The digestion of proteins and triglycerides begins in the stomach, as does the complex process of absorbing vitamin B12 and the defence against microorganisms through the action of hydrochloric acid.

The most important enzyme present in the stomach is pepsin, the function of which is to break the molecular chains of proteins, transforming them into smaller pieces. Pepsin is produced in cells first in an inactive form as a precursor: to be activated it requires the presence of acid, and this the stomach supplies.

The process requires a precise calculation of time and of costs. Intelligently, the acid is produced and the pepsin activated when there is food in the stomach, thus unleashing the digestive process. This arrangement increases the protection of the mucosa and reduces the risk of reflux.

### The "Witch's Brew"

The stomach's capacity to generate hydrochloric acid can reach industrial levels. A piece of metal can be dissolved by gastric juice, and plastic immersed in it melts within hours. It is like a witch's brew that converts steak into cream and kills all the bacteria and parasites that we inevitably swallow.

The stomach's acid is tremendously abrasive: it burns and destroys all that passes through. All of us have experienced moments of reflux, or even worse vomiting, when we taste the intensity of our own acid. This hydrochloric acid serves us as a liquid shield; it is essential for life, a powerful arm that defends us or attacks us when it is displaced from its natural environment.

I work with patients who suffer disorders in their eating behavior. The majority have a set of symptoms known as *bulimia* (the act of voluntarily vomiting after eating a large meal and/or binge eating). Normally, this conditions affects young women who have developed the pathological habit of vomiting daily, even several times a day, over years or decades. Bulimia is a psychopathological consequence of a lack of affection or of a psychological trauma that hasn't been resolved. It is a mental "trap" expressed in a love-hate relationship with meals. What happens to people who suffer from bulimia? Because of the frequent vomiting of bulimia, the gastric acid destroys the person's teeth; it dissolves them literally little by little until they break as if they were made of porcelain. The sufferer also gets severe dermatitis and ulcers on the fingers (which they use to provoke the vomit) because of the daily contact with hydrochloric acid. The vocal cords, the pharynx, the tongue, and the mouth are permanently inflamed and sensitive; and the lips and the corners of the mouth develop dry, hard skin. All this is without mentioning the damage done to the esophagus and the esophageal sphincter.

Fortunately, our digestive mucosa—and human tissues, in general—have an impressive capacity for regeneration. With care, they can be helped to recover and renew themselves, in spite of serious damage. Motor and muscular functions, however, take much longer.

Thankfully, the stomach is well protected against itself. A thick layer of mucosa, secreted by other cells in its walls, covers the interior and prevents it from digesting itself. If there is too much acid, or if the mucosa layer is deficient, the acidic content erodes the walls of the stomach and makes holes in it, leading to *gastric ulcers*. The production of a thick, resistant alkaline mucous is an exclusive characteristic of the cells of the stomach.

How does the stomach empty itself? It activates a system of nervous and hormonal control. The pyloric sphincter valve, located at the exit from the stomach, relaxes at intervals to let part of the chyme pass into the duodenum, the first part of the small intestine. The arrival of partially digested food in the duodenum unleashes the production of the hormones *secretin* and *cholecystokinin*, which stimulate the gallbladder and the pancreas and neutralize the stomach acid, alkalinizing it.

In summary, everything is designed to work together, with everything in its appropriate place and in the proper order, as organized by our digestive intelligence.

## Emotions and the Stomach

Important links can be found among the emotions, our psychoemotional condition, and our digestive state. Indeed, during ancient times, digestive difficulties were already beginning to be associated with psychological problems and the influence of the mind over the stomach was taken into consideration in the practice of medicine.

We all know that the stomach closes in a fist or a knot in situations of fear, grief, stress, or sadness. We lose our appetite because of emotional tension and when we fall in love. The stomach can be "broken" more than the heart. We note "an emptiness" or "a chill" in the stomach when we are lonely, abandoned, or deeply frustrated. We may say that we have "butterflies in the stomach" on receiving a pay raise or other great news or in a situation where we receive personal recognition for something we have done. Some of my patients tell me, "My stomach is full of anger." Others manage to locate "anxiety, suffering, hate, and rage" in it. Some people confess, "I haven't got the stomach for this," when they are talking about an intense or important event, or when they must make an emotional decision or change. Sometimes they tell me, "Doctor, my stomach is asking me only for sweets." The stomach can "open with anxiety, like a black hole without limit or bottom," and you can start to put everything in it that you find, especially sweets and junk food, trying to "quieten it or satisfy," this "false hunger … which in reality is a lack of happiness, peace, relaxation."

In the previous chapters, we have seen that we call this a "psychosomatization" of the emotions: the way in which situations are processed by our gut brain and expressed with and through sensations in our stomachs and intestines.

## Stomach Problems and Complementary Medicine

We will deal with two common gastric dysfunctions—*gastroesophageal reflux disease (GERD)* and *hiatal hernia*—in specific chapters later on. For the moment, let's focus on other common stomach problems.

### Helicobacter Pylori Bacterial Infection

This bacteria was identified in 1982 and is commonly seen accompanying gastritis (inflammation of the stomach lining) and gastric ulcers. Once confirmed and diagnosed, H. pylori infection has to be treated with antibiotics. In my professional opinion, antibiotic treatment must be done in a disciplined way, and the entire course of antibiotics must be taken in order to be most effective. This bacteria is very resistant and can cause major health problems. It needs to be treated thoroughly.

Once the bacteria have been eradicated with the correct course of antibiotics, it is essential, from the point of view of integrative medicine, to implement a two-month treatment of probiotics (food supplements of beneficial bacteria) in order to restore the intestinal microflora, because antibiotics destroy the "friendly" bugs as well as the bad ones. It is also worth considering carrying out a liver detoxification as a followup to the antibiotics. The patient also needs to follow a personalized dietary and naturopathic prescription.

There is little evidence in medical literature of the usefulness of natural treatments for H. pylori bacterial infection. We are still looking for methods that are truly effective and have long-lasting results. There is a promising study from Japan on the use of natural essences of certain plants and a combination of seaweeds. This seems to be an interesting alternative for the treatment of the bacteria. In my clinic, we keep up to date with the latest studies in this field and their results.

The herbal traditions of central Europe include recommendations for the treatment of this infection with strong herbal liqueurs made from sempervivum (houseleek), St. John's Wort, marigold, aloe, and honey. These liqueurs have to be taken in small doses on an empty stomach and this makes them of very limited application, except perhaps during holidays, when you can start each morning with a strong shot of alcohol.

## Gastritis

Gastritis refers to an inflammation of the internal gastric surface (mucosa), and it requires careful and prolonged treatment. To gain lasting relief, you will have to begin by sticking to a strict diet, preferably an alkaline diet that you keep to for at least a week. Such a diet involves eating frequently—every four or five hours—which means making five to six mini meals a day. You must eat small portions, all in the form of creams, purées, soups, juices, and porridges. Food must be kept plain and steamed, boiled, or cooked in the oven. Avoid spicy and fatty foods and sauces, all red vegetables, and limit fruit to two pieces a day. Meat and fish must be ground up in balls or stewed. You must eat lots of green vegetables (which are alkaline), boiled or puréed and not raw (except as juices). You need to limit pasta, wheat, and cereals (except as porridge). At the end of one week, other textures and flavors can be added to the diet, but always avoiding strong, spicy, or processed foods.

In natural medicine, the potato is highly regarded for its alkaline properties, which makes it calming and healing. When you suffer from gastritis, potatoes are a good thing to eat, in the form of purée after being either boiled or baked. An old and very effective remedy is fresh-squeezed potato juice. Drink 150 milliliters on an empty stomach. It is best to use organic potatoes. You can often find prepared potato juice in a health food shop.

I can confirm from my own experience that this is very effective. At the end of my time at high school, I got gastritis with spasms, typical for an adolescent at exam time. The treatment I was given was potato juice, along with a special diet. Obviously, at that age I didn't like this much, but the taste wasn't disagreeable and the truth is, drinking it on an empty stomach, it helped me get a little better each day. Each morning, my father took the trouble to grate two organic potatoes and to squeeze them immediately using a clean piece of muslin. I had to drink it rapidly, because the juice quickly forms a sediment and goes brown because of its high starch content. It is true that drinking potato juice required an effort on my part, but it left my stomach in perfect condition and I have some good memories of this little family morning ritual.

Porridge, the typical British breakfast dish made by simmering milled, fast-cook porridge oats in water or milk for around five minutes, has a relaxing and calming effect. (Note: If you want, you can use Irish steelcut oats, or pinhead oats, which are the whole oats but require much longer cooking.) Porridge regenerates the stomach mucosa and provides an excellent nutritional and energetic boost. The addition of a teaspoon of olive oil and a few dried plums offers both an original taste and increases the nutritional and curative properties of the porridge.

The pulp of aloe vera, extracted from the fresh plant, taken before the main meals, is another star remedy.

Infusions of sage, thyme, marigold, chamomile—or a mixture of these plants—drunk before and after every meal, relieves stomachache and regenerates the mucosa.

## Stomach Spasms

Whether caused by emotions on inflammation, stomach spasms can be relieved by sipping a strong, hot infusion of peppermint leaves. Many studies back the effectiveness of peppermint in reducing tension in a spastic stomach and relaxing the muscles of the digestive system. In the case of a "knot" in the stomach, or spastic ache, you can take three drops of essential oil of peppermint (the natural product at a therapeutic grade, from a specialized supplier) mixed with half a teaspoon of sugar. You have to dissolve this slowly in your mouth and breathe deeply. Note: It is important not to take the essential oil alone, but always with sugar or honey.

*I want to thank Irina for the great help she has given me in curing my thyroid nodules and in greatly improving my health, letting me feel young again, and full of energy and optimism for my personal and professional development; and above all allowing me to take care of my four year old daughter and watch her grow with happiness. Irina is a great practitioner with much wisdom and intuition who finds solutions to problems beyond the reach of traditional medicine.*

— *ROSA DE LA TORRE*, PHD, RESEARCHER IN SPACE SCIENCES, DEPT. OF THE OBSERVATION OF THE EARTH, NATIONAL INSTITUTE FOR AEROSPACE TECHNOLOGY, SPAIN

# 6

# The Small Intestine –
# A Tennis Court
# Hidden in Your Gut

When the food (or more exactly what is left of it) is dispatched from the stomach, its next destination is a long extremely twisted tube called the *small intestine*. The word small is a misnomer. If we were to stretch out this hosepipe, it would reach to 8–9 m (26–29 ft) in length with an average diameter of 3 cm (1 in). This is somewhat similar to the hosepipe in your garden: look and you will be surprised at what is in your gut, sharing space with many other organs.

The small intestine is a very special organ, being one of the most complex and perfect creations inside the human body; it is a biocomputer installed in the gut, which has been continually keeping its programs running for millions of years. The small intestine is in charge of our entire system of nutritional and energetic support, and of our defences through the immune system and our emotional balance.

The small intestine is large and that gives it the maximum ability to efficiently absorb nutrients. The ephithelium that makes up the walls of the small intestine is composed of three successive levels:

- The mucosa membrane forming epithelial folds
- Thousands of villi, or projections, designed to maximize surface area for nutrition
- Microvilli, tiny hairs that cover the villi, as seen in figures 1 and 2 on the next page

The wall of the small intestine looks as if it's covered with velvet, or else like the dense bristle of a brush; it is this that makes it the largest organ in the human body. Were we to spread it out in two dimensions, smoothing out all its folds, all its villi and microvilli, it would cover an area of 300 square meters (3,200 sq. ft). There is a whole tennis court hidden inside your gut! Thanks to the extent of its surface area, this small intestine is able to be in contact with everything that passes through the digestive system.

FIGURE 1

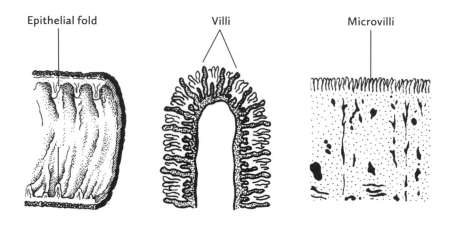

Epithelial fold       Villi       Microvilli

FIGURE 2

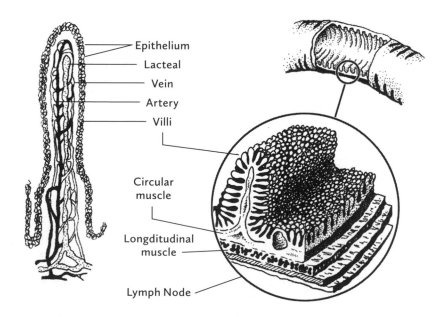

Epithelium
Lacteal
Vein
Artery
Villi

Circular
muscle

Longditudinal
muscle

Lymph Node

Everything that passes through this magically compressed space comes from the outside, and during its journey it will be processed, absorbed, and transformed into the building blocks of our body.

As mentioned earlier, the small intestine is also our body's principal "customs service," represented by operatives known as *crypts* (see figure 2). Each crypt is entirely self-supporting and consists of specialized epithelial cells, connective tissue, and immunocompetent cells (cells specialized in defending the body); it also has a small artery, a vein, a branch of the nervous system, and a lymphatic vessel.

## Strange Names

The small intestine consists of three consecutive parts: the *duodenum,* the *jejunum*, and the *ileum*. The word duodenum comes from the Latin *duodenum digitorum*, so called because anatomists of old declared that it measured 12 widths of a digit, or finger, that is around 18 centimeters (7 in). The word jejunum derives from the latin *jejunus,* or "fast" (in the sense of going without food). It was thus called because during autopsies (the medical examination of a corpse) medieval doctors always found this portion of the intestine "empty." The word ileum comes from the Greek and means "that which twists," so called because of its complicated route and shape. The ileum is the final part of the small intestine, the place where the most of the *lymphoid tissues* (Peyer's patches) are found. These are accumulations of immune cells, the most important part of our defence against infection and the development of disease.

## Where Does Your Cholesterol Come From?

Once inside the small intestine, the food is submitted to a bombardment of enzymes from the pancreas and liver. There are a few things that the pancreatic juices (the enzymes of the pancreas) can't digest. These are very powerful and abrasive and produce a strong "liquidizing" effect, breaking up everything that gets in their way. Bile is the juice of the liver and an essential part of digestion; it is a vital elixir that transforms all molecules of fat, good or bad, into soluble particles capable of passing through the "customs" of the intestinal lumen.

The digestion and absorption of fats is a very delicate, complicated process, and it is normally the first operation that fails. For this reason, a person may begin to have difficulties in digesting fats, his level of cholesterol may rise, and a scan may show that he has a fatty liver.

Contrary to popular belief, 70–80 percent of cholesterol, an important lipid molecule, is produced inside us in the liver, rather than from what we eat, and is essential to good health, when we keep it in a healthy limits. It is the main constructive material for our cell membranes and is a precursor in the manufacture of important steroid hormones in the body and bile acids. And it helps us assimilate vitamins A, E, K and D. We eliminate excess of cholesterol with the bile that is expelled by the gallbladder. My patients sometimes ask me, "If I don't eat fats, have a healthy diet, take exercise, and I'm thin, why have I got a high level of cholesterol?" A sizeable percentage of people who have had high cholesterol levels for a long time probably owe this to genetics or family history. In such cases, medical control and treatment of the condition is essential.

In the majority of cases, however, the reason is a dysfunction in digestive and metabolic processes, meaning that the small intestine, together with the liver, retains, reabsorbs, and recycles too much bile acid with cholesterol. It is an interesting subject for study with the aim of differentiating the causes.

As we have seen, bile participates in the digestive process inside the small intestine. At the end, some (lesser) portion of the cholesterol and of the bile salts will be captured by the cells of the ileum, reabsorbed, and returned to the liver. This is a normal process of recycling with no impact on health, because the rest (the "larger" part) goes to the colon and is eliminated with the feces.

When digestive enzymes and bile don't enter the small intestine in time and in adequate quantities (because of problems with the liver, gallbladder, pancreas, or something else), digestion is disrupted, food cannot be broken down correctly to be absorbed, and the nutritional contribution to the body is reduced. For example, if bile doesn't reach the small intestine sufficiently, hardly any lipids are absorbed and can cause diarrhea or constipation and bloating.

If badly processed and half-digested foods pass in this form to the colon, the billions of bacteria present there devour them in an unexpected feast with "fireworks" and "special effects." The production of gas increases, you feel swollen like a balloon, and the intestinal transit can be altered, leading, in one extreme, to episodes of diarrhea or, in the other direction, to constipation. The processes of putrefaction and bacterial fermentation begin to predominate. This is one example out of many of what can happen inside the intestine.

## The Intelligent "Border Guards"

In spite of its vital functional importance, the mucosa of the small intestine (its multiple folds facing out into the lumen) is very thin. In reality, it has the thickness of a cell and the delicacy of a piece of silk cloth. This gives it a high degree of selectivity over the transportation of adequate new nutrients to the rest of the body, but also a sensitivity and fragility toward chemical substances, toxins, and an excess of food. It is like a special division of cells—a line of soldiers without reinforcements who are obliged to maintain their ranks as determinedly as they can, putting up with a tour of duty from three to five days before replacements arrive. The mucosa reproduces itself (relines itself) completely approximately every five days.

As I said, it is a very fine material but it is "well stitched." The connections among the cells of the small intestine are very strong. Curiously, it is easier to harm or break the cells themselves than the connections among them. These "soldiers" are literally stuck to each other shoulder to shoulder and do not allow breaches between them unless they fall in battle. This, primarily, keeps us whole, so that we do not lose fluids or vital essence and do not leak little by little into the pipes of our digestive tract (this is exactly what happens in the cases of acute and serious gastroenteritis).

For nutrients, the only way into our "territory" is to penetrate (with permission previously given) the membrane of the cells of the small intestine, navigate through its cytoplasm (the liquid inside the cell), reach the farther shore of the same membrane and, once there, to be picked up by the bloodstream. Each of the nutrients is accompanied by an "official," a control undertaken by our own "transporter proteins." That is to say that there are no bridges or chaos, and all transport is by "ships" passing through customs with its rigorous system of control. Through this process we receive our fuel and energy.

If any food, chemical substance, toxin, or bacteria does not pass the control and is left without a visa, a "bouncer" immediately appears (a special, large cell belonging to the immune system). It collects the identification marks of the suspect (to add to its immunological database) and eliminates the intruder. From this moment on, every molecule similar to the aggressor will be automatically attacked by the "bouncer."

## Leaky Gut and Where It Leads

Situations in which the mucosa of the small intestine is seriously affected by exposure to toxins, certain chemical substances, bacteria or viruses, or general reduction in the body's defences can lead to a disorder known as *leaky gut syndrome*.

Breaches appear—holes caused by the loss or weakness of cells—and suddenly the frontier opens and everyone can cross it. The immigration service is overwhelmed because of lack of local control. Large sections of food molecules and fractions get into the bloodstream; instead of letters entering it, as it were, whole words or paragraphs get through. This produces a general alert. The immunological command center begins to produce troops of antibodies (the blood's defensive cells) to combat the trespassing agents and also records the characteristics of each "invader" in order to be able to attack it quickly the next time. It is an exaggerated and mistaken reaction directed against the foods that have passed through the mucosa of the small intestine. It causes the development of certain alimentary intolerances, and you begin to be "allergic" and sensitive to certain foods.

This is a provoked state corresponding to a particular situation. Food intolerances are not permanent allergies, rather they are passing sensitivities that need to be diagnosed and treated. Fortunately, modern medicine gives much attention to this disorder. There are many clinical scientific studies of leaky gut syndrome and its consequences for health.

A food intolerance means that we do not receive the nutrients of certain foods, and the arrival of these foods creates a "political conflict" within the intestine because they are "temporarily not wanted." The consequences are bad digestion, poor nutrition, and an immunological tension that reduces the body's general defenses.

There are many publications in the United States detailing the pathological links between leaky gut syndrome and illnesses such as psoriasis, atopic dermatitis, bronchial asthma, and multiple allergies. Some interesting and promising studies are emerging that show pathophysiological connections between leaky gut syndrome and chronic, degenerative autoimmune diseases. If the breaches in the small intestine persist, the immunological alert system is overloaded and pathological autoimmune reactions occur—in effect, the body begins to produce antibodies against its own tissues.

This is a new challenge for modern medicine, demanding an integrative overview that takes into account all of the factors that create immunological confusion and help sustain it. In today's medicine, we apply more complex treatments, which not only deal with symptoms but also aid the recovery of the whole of the intestinal mucosa and involve personalized nutrition.

If you want to know if you have any kind of food intolerance that may be causing you problems, the best thing to do is to take a full test and have the laboratory look for the presence of antibodies produced against each of the foods in question. This is a costly and complicated test, unfortunately, but it is reliable as it analyzes your blood and your antibodies. Individual tests for the most common foods, such as wheat, are available at a lower cost and may not need a doctor's note. Check with labs in your area.

When you receive the results of the test you will have to eliminate from your diet any foods to which you have been shown to have an intolerance for a period of six months. This is a sufficient period of time to erase the "erroneous" immunological memory from your body, eliminate the undesirable antibodies, and regrow the mucosa of the small intestine. I recommend you do all this under the supervision of a doctor.

If you can't afford to get tested, I suggest you begin with a detailed observation of your diet and keep a food diary where you note any foods that you suspect are producing any kind of digestive problem. When you have identified the "suspects," eliminate them from your diet completely for a period of 10 days and then reintroduce them one by one and observe the reaction of your digestive system or the response of your principal illness. Again, for your own safety, I recommend that you are examined and monitored by a medical professional specializing in digestive complaints (gastroenterologist).

> *Of the three "membranes of life" through which a human being interacts with his environment, the skin, the respiratory system and the digestive system, the last is the most complex and fascinating as much for its extent as its numerous functions. We shouldn't forget that it acts as a "second brain," given its great riches of nerve cells capable of secreting neurotransmitters, and that it is our primary immune system because of its size.*
>
> *This book by Dr. Irina Matveikova sheds more light on this authentic "intestinal ecosystem, and I can safely say it will be of great use both to professionals and to the general public. Congratulations!*

— *DR. JOSE HERNANDEZ MARAVER, DIRECTOR MADRID ANTI-AGING MEDICAL CENTER AND DIAGNOSTIC CLINIC*

# 7

# The Colon and Toxemia

A round eight hours after a meal, the remains of the food we have eaten leave the small intestine and go through the door called the *ileocecal valve* into the colon, or the large intestine. Whatever we have eaten has gone through a rigorous control and has been manipulated by our enzymes to such a point that everything necessary and nutritive has been absorbed and classified. The residue of lesser importance is transferred to the colon. It only has to go through a last phase before being "liberated" and expelled in its final form.

What happens inside the colon is far removed from the exclusive and clean neighborhood and environmental perfection of the small intestine. It is instead an overpopulated universe filled with billions of bacteria (as well as the fungi, yeasts, worms, and other parasites that can often be found here). It is a chaotic, unstable melting pot. Every microorganism is engaged in an almighty survival of the fittest, struggling to maintain existence, with its environment and source of nutrition subject to a permanent state of gang warfare. To give you an idea, it is like being forced to move from a chic neighborhood to a slum.

The remains of the food still have some value, including water, fiber, B vitamins, and precursors of vitamin K. As it enters the colon, it is attacked by all of the residents. Some ferment sugars, producing an abundance of "bubbles," while others—the good guys—take care of the fiber so that we can use it to feed our cells. A third group feasts on any residual proteins that it finds, generating toxic gas.

The final destination of a piece of cake, steak, or other food depends on the "Match of the Day" played by this hungry biomass—and which of the groups of bacteria will win out because of the strength of its army. This extended, multinational "society" of bacteria that occupies the colon is in no way a state based on order and social justice. It is instable and always exposed to change and shifting influences. It reminds me of Gulliver in Lilliput: we are enormous beings that have inside us universes of very intelligent Lilliputians. We can work with them and live in peace, or we can fight with each other. Indeed, in this particular universe, it's the little ones who very often win the fight!

Approximately 50 percent of the weight of the feces is made up of bacteria and the sub-products of their activity. The next time you look at your feces, remember that half of what you see has nothing to do with you or your food; it is a living mass full of bacteria—either peaceful cohabitants or invaders, depending on the state of your intestinal ecology.

The large intestine begins in a wide "bag" called the *cecum,* to which the appendix is connected, and terminates in the rectum. A healthy colon measures 1.6–2.5 m (5–8 ft.) long and reaches a diameter of 6–12 cm (2–5 in.). From the cecum to the rectum, the colon follows a series of curves that form a frame around the loops of the small intestine.

The second portion of the colon is called the *ascending colon*, a "hard-working" stretch of tube that has got to move its contents with more muscular force, pushing upward against gravity. Coming up against the inner face of the liver, it turns and becomes the *transverse colon*, the only organ that crosses the human body in a perpendicular direction from right to left, crossing in front of the stomach.

On reaching the extreme left, at the height of the spleen, the colon makes a narrow and complicated flexure and heads downward. From here it is called the *descending colon*. It has a different name in its final part, the *sigmoid colon,* because it is in the form of a fat "S." At the end, the colon reaches the rectum, and finally the anus.

The circular muscular layer of the colon is much fatter and stronger than its counterpart in the small intestine. The internal surface of the colon is lubricated, in most part, by a mucus secretion, which eases the passage of blocks of fecal material.

In the large intestine, there are no villi or microvilli, and its glands do not secrete digestive enzymes. The inside surface of the colon is formed by bulbous bags called the *haustra*. This word comes from the Latin *claudere*, from which comes the word *cloister*. Inside, the haustra are indeed very similar to semi-enclosed cloisters: they take in residues and become distended in order to accommodate a large amount of fecal material. In turn, this structure, which looks like a sausage from the outside, facilitates the muscular function of the intestine, generating waves of gentle movements every 20 minutes.

## Not a Garbage Bag

The large intestine is not a garbage bag. It is an organ that carries out several important functions, including the following:

- The secretion of *mucin*, a substance that lubricates the feces and facilitates their passage through the rectum and anus.
- Digestion. The bacteria in large intestine process food residues and fibers. This material is used to feed the intestinal cells.
- The absorption of water and part of the glucose, sodium chloride, and medications taken as suppositories. In the cecum and ascending colon the fecal

matter is almost liquid. It is here that the majority of water is reabsorbed, along with certain dissolved chemical substances.

- The excretion of calcium, iron, and medications.
- The formation of a healthy ecology via intestinal microflora, which provide the body's immune defenses.

These are all the good things that the large intestine does. On the other hand, as it is a recipient for residues and a universe for billions of bacteria, the colon can transform itself into a time bomb that can explode into the symptoms provoked by a high level or toxicity, or unleash a cancerous illness.

Like the small intestine, the large intestine has very few pain receptors, except in the area of the rectum and anus. There are few ways for the central nervous system to inform us about damage and pain. It is as if our intestine were mute (or almost so); it cannot shout to us about its suffering. For this reason, colon or bowel cancer is called a silent illness, given that its growth is not announced through pain until it becomes sufficiently advanced to block the intestinal passageway or cause bleeding. In many cases, the diagnosis of cancer of the colon is made in an advanced, late phase of the illness.

Pain receptors may be missing in the colon, but the rectum and anus are very sensitive and highly capable of producing painful sensations, to the point of being unbearable. This is because they are wrapped in a dense network of nerve receptors. This network can generate sensations ranging from pleasure (during a healthy expulsion of stools) to searing pain caused by the presence of anal fissures or hemorrhoids (piles). Both feelings can be very intense.

The anal canal is 5 cm (2 in) long. There are two anal sphincters, internal and external. The inner sphincter normally remains contracted to prevent any loss of feces through the anus. The exterior anal sphincter is subject to a high degree of control by the voluntary nervous system. The area of the rectum and the anus is irrigated by a circulating network of blood vessels including two extensive venous plexuses (a collection of veins clustered together). The drainage system of this area has no valves. An increase in tension and pressure in this area (such as from too much sitting or from straining to defecate) causes the veins to fill with blood, dilate, and swell, giving rise to the formation of internal or external hemorrhoids.

## The Journey Through Your Gut May Be Complicated

In reality, the shape and path through the body of the colon can vary greatly from that shown in anatomical diagrams. Many factors can influence the form and position of the colon. For example, the drawings on the following pages illustrate different routes

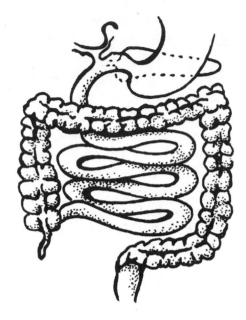

FIGURE 3

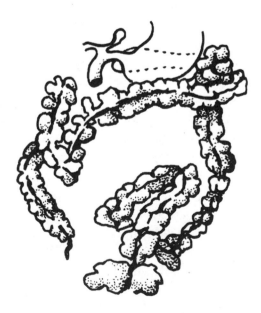

FIGURE 4

of the colon from the normal arrangement (figure 3) to an elongated and torturous variant (figures 4 and 5), and finally a spastic colon (figure 6).

The colon is an elastic organ that accommodates and adapts itself to circumstances. It can be lengthened, swollen, and even move its folds to unexpected areas within the very limited space of the abdomen. The tube of the large intestine can make an enormous amount of turns, as if it were tracing a goat path through the mountains. It can also be twisted and knotty. When it is overloaded and not contained within an adequate space, it can generate various types of symptoms—some false, others not.

Frequently, a megacolon or dolichomegacolon (an excessive and permanently dilated colon, long and twisted, with inadequate, weak muscle function) is an anatomic abnormality from birth, caused by a genetic and/or embryonic fault: there is often a family history behind this condition. I am currently treating a family for this problem. The mother is an old lady. She and her three daughters all have symptoms that indicate each has an enormous megacolon, twisted like a great python. X-rays show great similarities among their megacolons. However, the seriousness of their digestive disorders and other problems varies greatly.

One of the daughters, who takes great care of her diet, practices sports, and carries out periodic purges and colonic cleansings, enjoys good health and comes to my clinic just for maintenance. The mother and the older daughter, both overweight, with sedentary lifestyles and less careful about what they eat, complain of chronic fatigue, arthritis, constipation, and depression. The last daughter suffers from serious back pain and episodes of abundant and painful menstruation; she now knows that both complaints are made worse if she doesn't take care of her "monstrous" colon.

There can be a certain predisposition—the genetic inheritance of the family, which leads to a greater propensity to develop some kind of illness—but that does not mean you have to suffer from it. It depends on your diet and how well you take care of yourself.

I have many X-rays of patients with extravagantly shaped intestines. Sometimes the image of the abdomen is taken up by the colon alone—the entire space of the gut is occupied by what looks like an enormous inflated hosepipe. At other times, the spasms and muscular contractions produce an image similar to an hourglass or a cord. It would be interesting to exhibit them in a gallery so that people could become aware of the power and size of the contents of their abdomens.

In cases of excess weight and obesity, the folds of the intestine compete with fatty tissues and don't always win. A belly full of fat reduces the available space and limits the activity of the digestive muscles. This favors the retention of residues and increases the toxicity. People with abdominal obesity (those with large bellies) have a greater

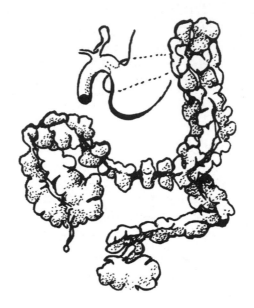

FIGURE 5

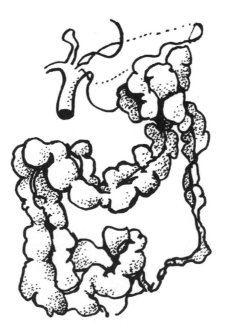

FIGURE 6

predisposition toward the development of colon cancer, and to suffering from exhaustion and fatigue and various types of degenerative illness.

## Intestinal Polyps

As mentioned above, the test known as a colonoscopy is a very important way to examine the colon. Normally, it gives a doctor information about the length and diameter of the colon, the presence or absence of polyps and/or diverticula, and about more even more serious problems. The same endoscopic process can be used to remove polyps and to take samples for detailed (microscopic) testing.

Today, colonoscopies are carried out on all people who have a family history of colon cancer, who have intestinal problems, and on everyone over 50 years old. It is a very important procedure in modern medicine for the prevention of cancer of the colon.

Another fantastic and very new way to study the colon is by means of a virtual colonoscopy, which displays the character and route of the colon in three dimensions. Twenty years ago, doctors couldn't even dream about this kind of technology now available to them.

A polyp is a visible growth, or protuberance, that projects from the surface of the mucosa and extends into the passageway of the intestine. Depending onto its microscopic characteristics, a polyp can be a lesion preceding cancer, as seen in figure 7 on the following page.

These growths appear more frequently in constipated intestines, where the environment is aggressive and the microflora out of equilibrium, or in conditions of irritation or chronic inflammation. The presence of genetic antecedents is also important.

Once a polyp has been diagnosed and removed, any recurrence can be prevented by the patient making serious changes to his or her diet, which will lead to improvements in the ecology of the intestine.

I know people who have annual colonoscopies, and each year they have polyps removed that have popped up inside them like mushrooms. This is itself is a sign of danger and a warning from the body that something serious and out of control is happening inside the cells of the intestines.

Primarily, it is important to take care of the transit through the large intestine: how long it takes for the remains of food to pass through the colon and be expelled. The slower the transit, the more toxic will be the feces and the worse conditions will be for the intestinal microflora. The contents of the residues are also important. Do they contain much fiber and vegetable waste or only proteins and the remains of processed meals? A transit that takes 24–36 hours is not considered alarming. If the exit of the residues takes a longer time (54–72 hours), it is an indication of an active process of putrefaction that can lead to toxemia.

To get an idea of the transit time of food through your digestive system, take three or four capsules of vegetable carbon (take separately from other medications) or any kind of food that changes the color of the feces, such as squid ink, for example (you will need to consume this in sufficient quantity). Note the time when you take the colorant and the time when your feces turn an intense black (in the case of the carbon). Then you can calculate the total time of the "voyage." Do this on a normal day and avoid taking a laxative at the same time.

The above is only a guideline to understanding the process, because the transit time will vary according to how much water you drink, your level of physical exercise, the rate of hormonal activity in your body, the quality of your meals, any stimulants you have taken, and the state of your emotions. Another factor is that large feces travel faster, given that their size makes the intestinal muscles work efficiently (*peristalsis*). Light feces that lack fiber are harder to transport. In addition, feces that take longer to travel absorb more water and become harder and more compact, making the act of eliminating them more difficult.

Poor functioning of the intestines causes the condition known as *intestinal toxemia*. This happens when the intestinal tract suffers as a result of an inappropriate diet, when the colon ceases to empty itself at the necessary times, when the digestive system has to process a course of antibiotics or other medications or adapt to the effects of chemotherapy or radiotherapy, and when detrimental bacteria replace the normal intestinal flora. It has been proven that toxification of the bowel occurs when the body absorbs too many residual toxins, and this is the cause of many disorders and illnesses today.

## Brain Activities and Intestinal Health

In earlier chapters we discussed the influence of a person's psychoemotional balance on the state of his or her intestinal health. It is beyond doubt that diarrhea, constipation, bloating, anal pain, and intestinal colic have an impact on psychological performance, intellectual capacity, and mood. These disorders, when they continue for some time, can determine the personality and behavior of the person who suffers from them.

To dig a little deeper into this subject, I would like to show how intestinal biology can affect mental activity and the most important cerebral functions.

AUTISM AND ATTENTION DEFICIT DISORDER (ADD): Behavioral disorders are largely manifestations of physiological problems inside our bodies. These include *autism* (a condition of mental development that affects the capacity of the individual to communicate, relate to others, and interact with the surroundings), *attention deficit disorders* (with or without hyperactivity), and other disabilities that do not lead to a definite diagnosis, as well as difficulties related to social interaction, communication, and a noticeably restricted repertoire of activities and interests.

There is no doubt that behavioral problems need to be tackled using a variety of scientific disciplines, and that they are almost certainly the consequences of various etiologies (origins and causes). Clinical studies and neurological and genetic hypotheses have contributed important data on this subject. Many researchers are trying to find explanations and solutions for these disorders because their incidence has been increasing for some time. In the developed world today, one child in every 166 is defined as autistic, whereas 50 years ago the ratio was 1 in 1,000. In certain parts of the United States, the incidence of autism is even higher, in some places reaching 1 in 82 children. The occurrence of attention deficit disorder (ADD, with or without hyperactivity), meanwhile is reaching epidemic levels.

How can a gastrointestinal disorder affect the brain and behavior? Some very intriguing hypotheses have been put forward. In children (and in adults) the fragility of the immune system or the lowering of the defenses leads to multiple infections, especially otitis (inner ear infections), colds, and respiratory problems, which are repeatedly treated with oral antibiotics. These drastically destabilize the intestinal flora and allow yeasts, fungi, and anaerobic bacteria to grow without control, colonizing the intestines, weakening them, and making them permeable, so that foods cannot be properly digested and assimilated. It may be that, despite their normal appearance, these children and adults are suffering from important deficiencies in nutrition.

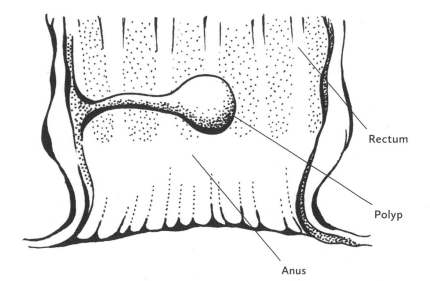

Rectum

Polyp

Anus

FIGURE 7

Badly digested foods pass through the porous barrier of the intestine (leaky gut syndrome), and once in the bloodstream they generate various alterations to the immune system: they overload it or suppress certain immunological functions, or else give rise to the "erroneous" creation of antibodies that attack the body's own organs and tissues (autoimmune disease). The fungi that infiltrate the damaged intestine and proliferate secrete toxins that confuse our defenses even more, and create a vicious circle of spiraling ill health. In this way, intestinal toxemia leads to auto-intoxication of the body and brain.

Certain undigested peptides and other toxic molecules that pass into the bloodstream through the permeable intestine can interact with the opioid receptors of the brain and block their normal functioning. Opioid receptors belong to the inner brain's group of proteins attuned to *endorphins* and *enkephalins*—molecules produced by the body that play an essential role in healthy brain chemistry and support cognitive functions, emotional stability, and psychological well-being.

When the work of the receptors that transport endorphins is impaired by toxins, important changes in mental, cognitive, and emotional activity can occur, including social isolation, stereotypical behaviors, radical changes of mood, misperception or insensitivity to pain, and changes to the senses of touch, sight, hearing, smell, and taste.

Many scientists maintain that the role of the gut, its high permeability, and the symptoms of toxemia, could be fundamental in the development of attention deficiency disorders and other behaviors. There are many clinical cases of improvements in the behavior of children when corrections are made to their intestinal microflora and digestive functions. It is not an absolute cure or solution, but it is an important factor that helps to improve and control their mental state.

In general, autistic children and the thousands of children with diagnosed hyperactivity or attention deficit disorder are born with immature and weak gastrointestinal systems. This is frequently explained by faults in embryonic development. More than 90 percent of these children have intestinal problems!

A first thing to look at is *intestinal dysbiosis*, an imbalance among the strains of bacteria inside the colon and an excess growth of organisms, especially of *candida albicans*, a yeast that causes fungal infections, as well as other fungi, yeasts, and parasites. The immune system in the majority of these children has very little capacity to act against these fungi, especially against candida, leading to imbalanced microbacteria in the colon that grow in a disproportionate way. The classic foods given to children—for the most part, wheat products, milk, sugar, and juices—can be very harmful to their intestines. In such cases, professionally supervised nutritional supplements and personalized diets are essential.

· · · · · · · ·

I remember an 11 years old girl. She was a patient who had suffered from constipation since birth. She had always been treated with laxatives and nourished with a lot of fiber: wholewheat products, a lot of cereals, milk, and fruit. At three years old, she was diagnosed with atopic dermatitis. She also had recurring breathing problems, which were frequently treated with antibiotics and antihistamines. As a consequence of this, at seven years old she was diagnosed with bronchial asthma, and to her treatment was added an inhaler and a low doses of corticosteroids. When she turned 11, she received another "stamp": attention deficit disorder with hyperactivity (ADHD) and they medicated her appropriately. This is a good example of a vicious circle.

Doctors have to act to address the symptoms and improve the health of this girl and they do it in a radical way, efficiently relieving the problems through the use of medications. Her parents, scared by the avalanche of problems, follow all the advice they are given, and they are right to do so. The girl knows she is different and closes herself in her world; she is used to visiting doctors and taking handfuls of medications.

This situation is not simple. Where do you start? I would begin with the most simple and obvious, and from there proceed toward the more complex. For the moment, it is necessary to respect the medication and not take any brusque decisions. We're talking about small children who are already used to suffering. The way to begin is with intestinal hygiene, which means a radical change of diet, the adoption of new habits, measures to get rid of parasites, and a suitable long-term regime of nutritional supplements to feed the intestines and the brain. In a few months, with improvements made to her digestive functions and with the aid of adequate nutrition, her doctors will probably be able to reconsider her need for multiple medications and their doses. When permeability has been confirmed the next step is a diet or, better, a study of food intolerances.

Even when we don't know the distant causes of various forms of autism, and disorders of attention and behavior, we can do much for these children and adults: we can prevent them from falling into vicious circles by working hard to help them. The experience of hundreds of children shows that if we break the vicious circle, the manifestation of behavioral disorders, and with it quality of life for those involved, can be noticeably improved.

## Autointoxication Is a Result of Intestinal Toxemia

Scientists and researchers are convinced that the end products of putrefaction irritate the nerve endings in the intestine wall. Because of this irritation, anomalous nerve impulses bombard the corresponding segments of the spinal cord. When this happens, the organs in other areas of the body that are associated with these segments of the spinal cord are negatively affected. Toxins produced in the colon are absorbed by the bloodstream and taken to the liver, which is charged with filtering and deactivating them. As this is not an easy task, given the enormous quantity of toxic material that we normally have in us, the liver can only temporarily slow down the passage of toxins into the general circulatory system and deposit them in its own tissues or in the fatty tissues of the body.

As you know, many provisional actions and decisions can be transformed into more permanent arrangements that you never find the time to get around to dealing with. The same thing happens with toxins. Once deposited, they begin their destructive toxic work, waiting for that day when their bearer will think about living a better life. It is also possible that the toxins evade the detoxification process because of some functional or pathological underperformance of the liver.

Another "illegal" escape route is by way of a porous section that may appear in the mucosa of the colon (we have already talked about the high permeability of the gut in relation to the small intestine). Some toxins have a chemical structure unknown to the liver, while many others acquire formulas similar to substances occurring normally in the human body, such as hormones. Among toxic chemical by-products found in the colon we can mention *indole, skatole, hydrogen sulfide, fatty acids, methane gas,* and *carbon dioxide.* Some of these substances are very toxic and smelly; they give the feces their characteristic and disagreeable stench.

Studies demonstrate that indole is highly toxic and carcinogenic (that it causes cancer). When high levels of phenol (carbolic acid, the metabolite of the amino acid tyrosine) and indole are recorded, it is the certain indication of the existence of a possible intestinal putrefaction. Phenol is so extremely poisonous that it is used as a detergent. It is both a local corrosive and a systemic poison that can damage the intestinal epithelium as well as the cells of the liver and the kidneys.

Skatole is another alternate toxic product of the bacterial action of tryptophan. It causes changes to the central nervous system, leading to symptoms of depression. It is also found concentrated in great quantities in the intestine after a high consumption of protein accompanied by constipation. When there is too much skatole in the bloodstream, a person has bad breath. Skatole and indole are partly responsible for the characteristic smell of feces.

Hydrogen sulfide is another derivative of the fecal decomposition process carried out by "bad" bacteria. In comparative terms, it is as toxic as cyanide. It is not surprising, then, that this toxic gas irritates the intestinal epithelium. The irritation provoked by hydrogen sulfide can cause congestion and serious inflammation.

Mercaptan smells much like a gas leak in the home. In fact, suppliers of natural gas add a small quantity of mercaptan, so that a leak can be detected, given that natural gas is colourless and odourless. Mercaptan and other gas with a disagreeable smell are created in a putrefied intestine, and their uncontrolled and audible escape is usually a cause of shame.

Tyramine is a putrefied by-product of the breakdown of tyrosine. It is in charge of liberating the stress hormone norepinephrine in the body. Norepinephrine causes blood vessels to diminish, and this can lead to an increase in blood pressure.

We know that ammonia is one of the substances produced in the intestine by the action of proteolytic bacteria (which break up and consume protein residues). One of the functions of the liver is to convert this ammonia into urea, so that the kidneys can excrete it. When the liver isn't working correctly, the bloodstream has abnormally high levels of ammonia. As a result the level of ammonia in the cerebrospinal fluid increases, and this can cause serious neurological problems with psychological consequences.

Another very toxic substance, *clostridium perfringens enterotoxin*, is found in the residues of putrefaction characteristic of an intestine affected by constipation. Clostridium is a kind of pathogenic bacteria that has a minor presence and activity in a healthy colon but which can multiply and dominate a "blocked" colon. An enterotoxin is a specific toxin that affects the cells of the intestinal lining and that is conducive to the development of cancer of the colon.

As we can see, the role of microorganisms in the large intestine is very important for health. A balance in the intestinal microflora and regular muscular motility are needed to control the development of many pathological processes. The ability of the same bacteria to harm or benefit health demonstrates the importance of maintaining a balance among bacterial strains, their environment, and their nutrition.

Because foods constitute the principal source of toxins, the enormous importance of adapting our diet to our organic needs is obvious. Even healthy, natural foods consumed in excess can be a source of gut intoxication. When the food you eat is adapted to your ability to digest, burn, and eliminate it, there is no undesirable accumulation of toxins that can lead to the development of diseases.

I suggest you to take a little time to analyze the chart on the next page. At first sight it may seem complicated, but it isn't. It shows how a toxically overloaded and constipated colon can give rise to many disorders in the body and unleash the development of serious diseases.

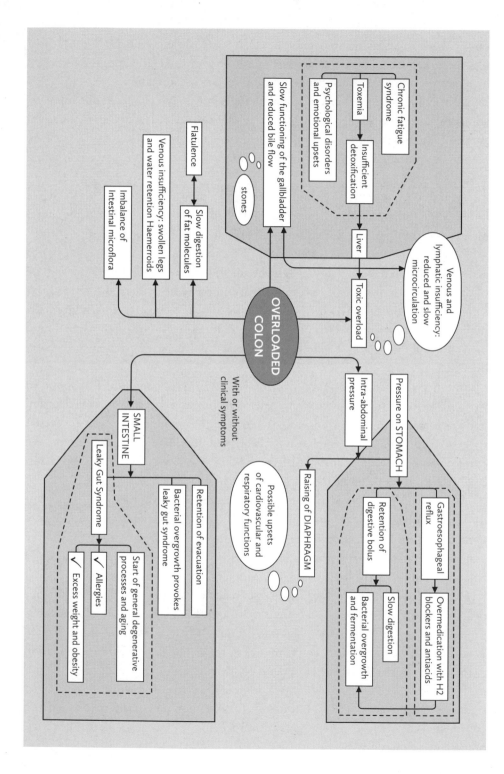

# 8

# Constipation:
# The Ever-Present Shadow

It is ironic that, despite widespread information about taking care of our exterior selves—keeping clean and staying healthy—we give little thought to the value of maintaining health and cleanliness on the inside. Many of us have childhood memories of enemas performed at home, though. Our grandparents knew how to take care of their intestines and their digestion.

Until I was eight years old, I spent almost every summer with my grandmother in a village of 10 houses lost in the woods. Twice a week, a cart would bring us bread, salt, and matches from the city; this was our only contact with the world. There was radio but no television; everything we had was fresh, homemade, and handcrafted.

My grandmother, it turns out, was a healer and knew all about medicinal plants and natural remedies. Instead of fairy tales, she told me stories about the powers and virtues of nature. Sometimes we would pick flowers together—stems, roots, and fruits—on long journeys through the woods. Her house always smelled of herbs, infusions, and oils. The kitchen, which had an enormous Russian chimney, was always full of jars and tinctures, and in the loft were hung bunches of various plants and flowers that she had dried there.

My favorite playthings were the fruits and vegetables in the garden, flowers, plants, bits of wood and, of course, my beloved pets. I would watch my grandmother preparing aromatic and curative remedies, and afterward, I would play at healer myself, trying to put bandages and compresses on my cat or trying to apply curative drops to the nose of the dog. I added infusions to the pig's food and created drawings on its enormous hide using different muds and dyes. The cow liked fresh plants, so I fed it a variety of combinations of medicinal herbs. I never managed to make friends with the geese. They were very big and quick, and they pecked my bottom whenever they could. Neither did I trust the bees; however, the chickens were charming and immediately ate the mixtures of roots and seeds that I offered them.

I was a delicate child, and when I lived in the city I was frequently ill. My summers were therefore filled with my grandmother's intensive treatments. I remember beginning the day with aloe vera pulp accompanied by a shot of some bitter extract.

Just thinking about it now, I get the same bitter taste in my mouth, recalling the interminable infusions that I took. Then there were the enemas that I considered an unavoidable punishment. I still have the image of the compresses, the ventouses (for cupping), the creams and pomades, and the inhalations. I also had to undergo a weekly ritual that consisted of a session in a sauna full of aromatic vapors, where my grandparents gave me typical massages using birch branches that had been previously heated and soaked in water.

Our diet, of course, was clean and natural and very healthful. It was enriched with fresh cheeses, curds, kefir, the obligatory juices (especially celery, carrot, and sauerkraut!), various pulses, honey, and recently baked homemade bread. The worst thing for me was the glass of milk I had to drink immediately after milking the cow: it tasted too "natural" to me.

I know the first years of my childhood were not normal, but I imagine that I may have prompted some nostalgic souvenirs of your own. This is a good moment to begin to rediscover things natural and authentic and incorporate them into our modern lives.

If the toilet or washbasin in your house is damaged, you naturally do not use it and you call a plumber. You wouldn't think of going into a toilet that was foul-smelling and full of stagnant water with excrement floating in it. What if no one comes to help you? Then you have to live in these extremely disagreeable conditions, knowing that you can't flush the toilet and eliminate the residues that have accumulated. Imagine your face when you are confronted with such a repulsive scene!

I am sure that in such a situation, you would react by throwing a bucket of water down the toilet (unless, that is, this merely raises the level of the stagnant "lake"), or else you would calling the 24-hour emergency services or asking for help from a friend. You'd be dead right to do so!

If you try to apply this solution to your blocked guts yourself, it won't work; you won't discharge the residues that have accumulated. You have to try to stimulate them from above or from below, without waiting too many days. Agreed? You just need to learn how to do it and what to use; each of us has his own digestive character and sensitivity to laxative remedies.

Approximately 70 percent of my current consultations are with people who in addition to different health conditions are suffering from chronic constipation. It is such a common and stubborn complaint, and so difficult to treat, that one day I think I will get all my patients together and found a constipation club (I'll probably look for a more attractive and sophisticated name). Then my team would be able to work with groups to help more people with their therapies, good humor, and various exercises. Reeducating people about good hygiene and diet, accompanied by psychological support, will be important parts of this work. If this appeals, come and join us and help me organize it.

Constipation is a personal, emotional, and social problem, as well as an economic one. Not only is it costly in terms of money spent on laxatives and visits to the doctor but also because of the serious consequences to health that chronic constipation brings, and the bodily toxemia it provokes. Only with a good diet and correct intestinal hygiene (I am referring to transit and microflora) can we prevent cancer of the colon.

Constipation is a very familiar condition: the majority of us have suffered from it on at least one occasion. In fact, recent research has demonstrated that one in seven people suffer from constipation. As well as being a relatively common complaint, it has become a social taboo. Often I am the only witness of this illness, in spite of the fact that the person tells me he has a partner, family, and friends.

We learn in childhood that the "stomach" can malfunction, and that if this happens you take a laxative. We all have memories of some constipated member of our family.

## Personality and Constipation

The connection between personality and constipation is interesting. This relationship is expressed through the enteric nervous system and the metabolism of serotonin, the hormone of well-being that in its turn stimulates intestinal motility.

It has been observed that individuals with chronic constipation usually have irritable personalities, are rigid in their ideas and concepts, and are difficult to live with. In contrast, people with a normal intestinal rhythm are usually more open, more relaxed, easier to live with, and more at ease with themselves. Researchers have shown that men can be hiding more than is apparent here, out of a certain insecurity about their intestinal habits. Men's productivity at work is reduced by twice as much as women's because of constipation, and men avoid using toilets at work more than women. Men joke about this problem in public, but when it affects them personally they are more likely to suffer in silence.

The constipated intestine, seen from a psychoemotional point of view, is an extreme manifestation of deep emotional suppression, terrible fear, and an unbearable degree of control. It also indicates low self-esteem, which leads to exaggerated perfectionism involving the setting of unachievable goals (but no one knows this: it is hidden in the gut). Emotions, passions, and hidden desires are stuck and lodged in the folds of the intestine, with no way for them to get out. People who are affected by this condition know little about losing weight, relaxing, and letting themselves be carried along by life; instead, they feel themselves to be constantly exposed to the judgments and criticisms of others. They have a tendency toward hypochondria, melancholy, and depression and can be prone to anxiety attacks; sometimes they eat compulsively, anxiously, and rapidly to fill themselves up.

When I meet a patient with a history of chronic constipation, I come face to face with all of this emotional baggage and physical suffering. Of course there are variations and exceptions to these generalizations.

Women usually suffer more from chronic constipation than men. Mostly when they seek medical help they have often been addicted to laxatives and suppositories for several years. The youngest of them can have small movements of the colon (producing few stools) once a week or once every 10 days, without taking any measures. Older women usually prefer to clean themselves out with laxatives every night.

The most representative group is composed of people who are very busy and speedy: super-responsible control freaks who are always connected to the world and have diaries full of things to do, both important and insignificant. They dedicate their lives to serving (and controlling) everyone around them while they forget or ignore the basics of life. They are normally well aware of their digestive problems, and have spastic intestines and disordered bowel movements; they frequently suffer from inflamed hemorrhoids.

They often drastically limit certain foods in their daily diet (fats, milk, pulses) in order to control their digestive disorders and bloating, gradually accepting a reduced quality of (digestive) life without being aware of the serious results this can have. Constipation is transformed into yet another obligation and something that must be forever controlled. These people can never allow themselves to forget to take something to go to the toilet because their guts will never ask them to expel their feces naturally, with gentle movements. Their tummies seem like traitors to them: mute, lazy, without emotions, and insufficiently communicative—except by means of gas and painful cramps due to an overdose of laxatives. They get the impression that their gut doesn't care whether it is fed fiber and all sorts of wholewheat products, or that they regularly visit the gym: it is just on strike. It is a strike that lasts a whole life.

How frustrating and draining it is, this permanent state of not feeling clean inside and always feeling bloated! Ironically, the husbands and partners of constipated women seem to experience the complete opposite: every morning they go to the toilet like clockwork. The first thing they do is have a good bowel movement, with great pleasure without problems; they do this religiously, with no sense of rush or pressure. This is impossible for the feminine mind to understand! More than this, it makes women cross: it has to be in the morning! It provokes feelings of anger, even hate.

Women, your men are not going to suppress their bowel movements out of solidarity with you, nor the pleasure they take in them. Nor are they going to hide their perfect intestinal functions. It makes no sense to get angry. The best thing to do is to learn from your significant other. I assure you that men are not more primitive—they are simply more able to concentrate on doing one thing at time (not 10). They know how to set priorities, and they tend to give precedence to the more corporal ones. In general, they never suppress the desire to defecate, sacrificing it because they are in a hurry. I repeat, in general—there are exceptions to everything.

And you? How many things are you thinking off when you go to the toilet? Where does your mind go to when the "mute" part of your body is looking into the toilet, without expression or emotion? Do you watch the clock? How much time do you have to move your bowels? "Not much, just a minute." Did you know that a healthy intestine moves at the speed of one centimeter (less than half an inch) per minute? The movements (peristalsis) of the colon are very slow and gentle and, as we have seen, it is a long tube. It cannot accelerate, except if you "hit" it with a laxative, then it spits out something hysterically, half loose and in a hurry.

Try to find 10–15 minutes to carry out a regular daily ritual of sitting down calmly and relaxed, ideally with a step or footstool beneath your feet. Try to stop thinking and concentrate on your belly, caressing it with a massage and breathing from the abdomen. Maybe it makes sense to get up a little earlier in the morning, to stretch your body, drink a glass of warm water or mint tea; two spoonfuls of olive oil in lemon juice can also be a great help in getting your digestive functions going. Organize your head, smile, and start the day with a bodily ritual, taking charge of your whizzing brain and fix it on "the here and now." Do this for three weeks. You will definitely see results.

What I'm talking about here is the classical approach to creating a conditioned reflex. In 1890–1900, this was studied by the famous Russian physiologist Ivan Pavlov, who got his dogs to develop required habits and digestive behaviors through repeated stimulation and memorization in the canine mind. Thanks to these experiments, Pavlov confirmed the laws of conditioned reflex. We are more complicated than dogs, but we know very well how to form conditioned reflexes. I have already pointed out that in infancy children learn perfectly about the times for eating, sleeping, or going to toilet; they are able to hold on and suppress their physiological stimuli, in spite of the fact that as newborn babies they were completely free from times and rules. Adults can relearn behavior; they can consciously and positively condition themselves.

*I am 42 years old. I have been constipated since I was little, and even when I was very young, 14 or 15 years old, I started to take laxatives to go to the toilet. I began by taking laxatives once a week. So if my intestines were already lazy, the use of laxatives made them worse. In fact, I could say that I only went to the toilet when I took laxatives. Both the dose and the frequency of taking the laxatives increased progressively, resulting in a daily abuse of them.*

*Tired and with little hope that my problem could have a solution, I went to see Dr. Irina who prescribed the cleansing of colon with hydrotherapy in four sessions. I also undertook treatment to clean my liver over a week. I took various probiotics with the object of regrowing my intestinal flora. Instead of taking laxatives, I was instructed to take a supplement of magnesium and water-soluble fiber. I have not gone back to taking laxatives.*

*The colon hydrotherapy has been truly marvelous, and I will continue to do it, following the recommendations of the doctor. Right from the first session you feel a sense of well-being that I personally had never experienced before. The reeducation of the habit of going to the toilet is slow; it doesn't happen overnight, and in my case to be able to count on the help of an expert in natural digestion has been a great help.*

*I have a 12-year-old daughter who has shown signs of constipation since she was little, and who often has problems and pains in her gut. Once, we even went to the emergency department thinking that she was suffering from appendicitis, when what was happening to her was that she hadn't been to the toilet for a long time. This episode was, in fact, what made me go to see Dr. Irina, about whom I had heard good reports. Following certain guidelines based on moderate changes to her diet over 30 days, taking certain dietary supplements, and the habit of sitting on the toilet each morning for a good bowel movement —these measures have completely changed the digestive behavior of my daughter. She has not had any more problems.*

— **P.**, BIOLOGIST, SPANISH NATIONAL CANCER RESEARCH CENTER

## What is Constipation?

When the feces are hard and infrequent (less than three times a week) and require great force to expel them, these are the symptoms of constipation. Constipation can cause pain on passing the feces and, if they are of great size, can break the mucosa membrane of the anus, which can cause it to bleed and possibly create an anal fissure. This condition can be accompanied by abdominal pains characterized by:

- Distension and flatulence, that implies the accumulation of gas
- a white coating on the upper part of the tongue
- headaches
- pain on defecating, hemorrhoids, and anal fissures
- halitosis (bad breath)
- bad body odor

Constipation is frequently caused by:

- Lack of foods rich in fiber and the abuse of animal proteins, refined products, fast food, sweets, and white flour.
- Food intolerances
- Dysbiosis, an imbalance in the intestinal ecology.
- Illnesses and upsets in the digestive tract above the colon (stomach, gallbladder, liver, pancreas, and small intestine)
- Dyskinesia and the presence of gallstones (lazy and distended gallbladder, retention of bile, and the formation of mud or bilious stones).
- Sedentary lifestyle and lack of exercise
- Inadequate (low) intake of liquids
- Delaying going to the toilet, or chronic suppression of the urge to defecate
- Stress and travel, producing spasms and muscular contractions in the intestine
- The presence of intestinal disease, such as irritable bowel syndrome, an inflamed intestine, cancer of the colon, diverticula disease (the presence of protuberances in the form of little bags in the wall of the colon), stenosis (a narrowing and rigidity of the intestinal walls), polyps
- Pregnancy
- Certain metabolic and hormonal conditions: diabetes, obesity, polycystic ovary syndrome, hypothyroidism. Hormonal changes that can happen during pregnancy, premenstrual syndrome, and menopause
- Mental health problems and neurological disorders
- Taking certain medications (codeine, analgesics, sedatives, iron, calcium antidepressants, tranquilizers, antacids) that reduce peristalsis (regular muscular movements of the gut) in the intestine
- Weakness of the abdominal wall muscles, of the diaphragm, and of the pelvic floor that play a part in defecation
- Genetic predisposition to constipation, congenital anomalies such as megacolon
- Illnesses of the anus and rectum, such as fissures and hemorrhoids, which make defecation painful and cause the patient to avoid or suppress all intestinal movements
- Age. Constipation is very common in people over 75, due to alterations in intestinal transit, aggravated occasionally by immobility and polypharmacy (taking multiple medications).

## The Treatment

Treatment needs to be personalized and holistic, based principally on educating the patient. A study of the colon (by means of a colonoscopy) is very important if the patient has a history of more than 10 years of constipation and is over 50 years of age. If there is a family history of colon cancer, a colonoscopy is essential. The removal of polyps during this endoscopic procedure can help control intestinal motility.

A natural treatment with probiotics and other supplements, undertaken after removing any polyps, as well as a corrected diet, can prevent relapse and impede the formation of new polyps. Fortunately, the use of probiotics in therapeutically high doses is increasingly accepted by conventional medical doctors specializing in the digestive system.

## Laxatives

Laxatives are the most commonly used medications in the struggle against constipation. The market in pharmaceutical laxatives is flourishing. It is estimated that more than 15 percent of the population of the United States, Canada, and the United Kingdom suffer from chronic constipation. Women are affected by constipation up to three times more than men. Among adults with constipation, 16 percent in Europe on average, 20 percent in the UK, and 40 percent in the US use laxatives. In the United States, approximately 38,000 tons of laxatives are sold each year, corresponding to $700 million annually. Understandably, only a minority of these people seek medical help for such a common, "squalid" complaint as not being able to move their bowels. There are almost certainly hundreds of thousands more people who suffer in silence.

I understand completely that taking laxatives is not done on a whim. It is the only method possible when the person doesn't know what else to do. Faced with a lack of information, and not having personalized attention and education on correct toilet hygiene, many people don't know that there are remedies that are quicker and more efficient.

Laxatives attack the mucosa of the colon, acting only in a symptomatic way, and their efficiency is very limited. They provoke spasms and stress in the colon, which allows only part of the accumulated materials to be evacuated. Laxatives only help clean part of the intestinal passage; they don't eliminate the heavy layer of mucous saturated with toxins that coats the colon.

The oral route of taking laxatives is the least desirable, because it can interfere with the digestive process and the absorption of nutrients and cause the patient to dehydrate.

People who suffer from constipation typically self-medicate with laxatives, but it is the worst way to solve the problem. The most commonly used laxatives, which are considered natural, are usually based on the principle of stimulating the nerves of the intestine with the aim of accelerating its peristalsis and causing spasms and semiliquid deposits. In the long run, though, they can lead to a tendency to retain feces, meaning that all they achieve is to create a progressive spiral by which the dosage is increased but the constipation gets worse.

As a general rule, because laxatives act as chemical irritants that stimulate the muscular walls of the colon and abnormally force it to expel the irritating substances, their continual use provokes irritation and inflammation of the intestinal walls. The brutal stimulation of the colon leads to *atony* (a lack of motility) of the intestinal walls and alters the normal rhythm of the organs of the digestive system, which in turn makes the constipation more serious. It is very easy to become dependent on laxatives, thereby destroying the colon's ability to self-regulate evacuation of the bowel.

One common mistake is to think natural is better—to go to a health shop and buy herbs, infusions, and natural laxative preparations thinking that, at least, these items will do you less harm. In fact, the most powerful and irritating laxatives are purgative medicinal plants. They should only be used one or two days a week or perhaps to purge yourself twice a month, and the rest of the time use other remedies and foods. If you use irritating laxatives on a daily basis, within two weeks you will be hooked on them and your bowel will become irritated and partially resistant, which will oblige you to increase the dose or to try other herbs.

If you take away the normal physiological function of any organ (even mildly), like a muscle it loses its tone, its capacity to react, and its elasticity. As with any convalescent who has been immobilized for a length of time and can't yet get about easily, the intestine has to recover its rhythm and strength little by little, and free itself from the dependence on laxatives. It is a long and difficult process, but the body will thank you in around two months. That is nothing, when you compare it to 20 years of being constipated, is it?

## Alternative Advice

As a first step, I recommend you give precedence to supplements composed of magnesium salts, alternating distinct formulations and always taking care not to abuse these substances but to respect your own sensitivity as far as the correct dosage. The most gentle of these are magnesium carbonate and magnesium hydroxide. Magnesium sulfate is stronger and more potent. Although these are food supplements and are not defined as drugs, you should always ask about their compatibility with any other medications you are taking at the same time.

Magnesium is a laxative that primarily acts to stimulate the muscular activity of the intestines and the gallbladder. It has no irritating local effects and has an antistress effect on the gut brain. It trains the intestinal muscles to work with regularity. To avoid the loose stools often associated with magnesium, it is best to combine this mineral with supplements of water-soluble fiber rich in prebiotics and inulin, such as psyllium and flax, and with probiotic supplements. You need to take fiber supplements separately (spacing them 1–2 hours apart) from other medication because the fiber can affect the absorption of the medications. Neither magnesium nor water-soluble fiber supplements lead to dependency nor do they alter the muscular tone of the intestines—quite the opposite, in fact.

Taking control of your bowel habits is an important first step in improving your gut health. It will enable you to get things on an even keel so that you can begin the work of devising a personalized diet, doing colonic cleansings, and creating the conditions for the intestinal mucosa to be restored to optimal health. These steps will help you balance the intestinal microflora in your colon and allow you to reeducate your body as to correct digestive hygiene.

The use of glycerine suppositories or commercial micro-enemas should only be occasional, for example when traveling. Used sparingly, suppositories can bring great relief, but I do not recommend that you use them every day. Remember that the anus is highly sensitive and has an abundant network of receptors connected to the nervous system. When you introduce a suppository (localized medication) into the anus, the chemical substances in it irritate and activate anal receptors and provoke a wave of muscular spasm, usually along the rectum itself. This causes you to rapidly expel any feces accumulated in the lower part of the colon, all in one go. This has nothing to do with a complete bowel movement. It is for only very occasional use, as a last resort. Moreover, if you continue to use suppositories, as with any laxative, it will start to take longer to produce the desired effect—the feeling of urgency that makes you want to evacuate the bowels. Suddenly, you find yourself waiting 15–20 minutes, then 30 minutes, and so on.

What has happened? The constant and frequent local irritation of the nerve receptors causes them to become desensitized, the mucosa grows hard because of the chronic irritation, and the natural reflex becomes disordered. Recovery time is then lengthened and complicates the therapeutic process. It is vital, therefore, to restore the gut's natural reflexes so that your body can return to functioning the way it is designed to do.

What is normal functioning in defecation? Well, when the final residues are ready to be expelled, the bolus of feces accumulates in the wide part of the rectum (which is called the rectal ampulla) and presses gently toward the exterior sphincter of the anus, waking up the nerve receptors and provoking the need to defecate. The prolonged abuse of suppositories deadens these nerve endings, so that your rectum may be warning you that the moment has arrived but the "alarm bell" no longer works because you have turned it off.

Natural alternatives to a local laxative include a home-administered enema, carried out gently, using a lukewarm infusion of filtered water and chamomile or thyme. Another effective method is to introduce into the anus 100–150 ml (4–5 fl oz) of virgin olive oil using a rubber "pear" that can be bought in a pharmacy and is normally used for cleaning the nostrils of a baby. Olive oil is a gentle muscular stimulant, an excellent lubricant, and has regenerative and anti-inflammatory properties. Once the olive oil has been introduced slowly into the anus, I recommend trying to hold it in the rectum for half an hour or more. It is best to be lying down and to relax. For some people I recommend doing it before going to bed so that you can have a bowel movement in the morning. This is a good method for preventing anal fissures and bleeding hemorrhoids. The olive oil helps retrain the colon and restores the ritual of having bowel movements in the morning; however, it does not clean the tract of the large intestine deeply and completely.

One very important point to make is that when the muscular tone of the intestine is reduced, consuming fiber provokes a significant distension of the colon yet does not lead to the muscular movement necessary to evacuate the bowel. This is very uncomfortable and confusing, because everyone recommends that you eat fiber for a healthy bowel, but doing so may lead to just feeling bloated.

At my clinic, I personalize your treatment, including prescribing specific types of fiber you should be using for your particular digestive problem, and I also explain in detail the difference between the types of fiber. For example, there are times when we are constipated when consuming a lot of grains, particularly wholewheat products, actually increases irritation in the gut and causes bloating without facilitating intestinal transit. Sometimes, therefore, it is better to begin treatment using water-soluble fibers that form a soothing gel in the intestines, such as psyllium seed husks and oats, in order to stimulate the muscular functions of the bile ducts and the intestine.

Laxatives vary considerably, too. Some only eliminate liquids and create loose stools; others lead to the passage of "goat droppings"; a third kind provokes embarrassing rumbling cramps.

Every gut represents a challenge, an apprenticeship. The gut protests; it shows its character of iron; it doesn't move unless you hit it with a laxative; and in spite of this it doesn't listen to you and insists you give it permanent attention. What kind of life is that? You could say: "I have always been that way; it is one of my characteristics." Okay, but this is not your original design nor is it by definition a disability.

I urge you to take action to restore the health of your gut. Perhaps one day, instead of a passing over this unimportant subject and taking a laxative yet again, you could also demonstrate that you have a will of iron, discipline, and sufficient patience to finally enjoy good health. One day I would wish to hear about some new foundation or institution that offer classes or courses to those patients who are recorded to have digestive problems, thereby fostering the motivation and personal (or economic) interest to attend such courses. I am certain that there is much to be gained—both on a personal level as well as in costs to our entire health system.

## Colonic Hydrotherapy

The physiopathological consequence of constipation is a saturated colon overloaded with toxins (intestinal toxemia). This creates an imbalance in the microflora of the intestine, greater permeability of the intestinal epithelium, and accumulation of toxins in the lymphatic system, liver, and blood that leads to various health problems and, over time, the potential for the development of chronic systemic illnesses and cancer of the colon.

Colonic hydrotherapy, followed by a balanced diet, probiotic supplements, and exercise, is an effective solution for the treatment of constipation.

Ridding the body of all toxic residues, hard feces, microorganisms, and excess mucus allows the colon to recover its healthy ecology, as well as its capacity to generate and maintain a healthy, functioning intestinal epithelium. The continual irrigation of the colon with water during a treatment directly stimulates the muscles of the digestive tract. This helps restore tone and motility in the intestine.

After the deep cleansing of the colon, it is important to establish a plan covering diet, supplements, and personal exercises that includes hygienic reeducation and psychological support in cases in which it is necessary. This therapeutic combination produces significant results.

### NUTRITIONAL RECOMMENDATIONS

By way of practical advice here is a list of foods and supplements that possess laxative properties and which stimulate intestinal transit. Many of them are not in common use, but they can be bought in health food shops.

- **PLUM JUICE WITH ITS PULP.** Drink a glass of the juice with breakfast.
- **STEWED PRUNES.** Cover 10 dried prunes with water in a saucepan and rehydrate by simmering in water for 5 minutes. Prunes can be eaten as dessert after dinner or as a snack in late afternoon.
- **STEWED APRICOTS.** Rehydrate 10 dried apricots and use as above.
- **ORGANIC BEETROOT JUICE.** Drink a glass of the juice with dinner.

- **SALAD OF COOKED AND GRATED BEETROOT.** Toss with olive oil and garlic (not mayonnaise) and eat a portion with dinner.
- **SAUERKRAUT JUICE** (fermented cabbage). Drink 2–3 tablepoons of the juice *before* dinner.
- **FLAXSEED DRINK.** Soak 2 tablespoons of flaxseeds in a glass of water for 8–10 hours, stir well, and drink on an empty stomach (the seed and the water). You can drink another glass at bedtime, if you wish.
- **VIRGIN OLIVE OIL.** Mix 2 tablespoons of oil with the juice of a fresh-squeezed lemon and consume 15 minutes *before* breakfast.
- **MASHED ALOE VERA.** Mash the pulp of a fresh leaf of aloe vera (without the skin) and consume two tablespoons *before* each main meal.
- **ORGANIC FLAXSEED OIL.** Take 1 tablespoon of the oil on an empty stomach and at night (you can use 2 capsules of flax seed oil). Note: keep the oil in the refrigerator as it will turn rancid from light and heat.

*It is a pleasure to write a brief comment for your book, as colleague and as your patient. Together, we have treated patients with nutritional disorders and consequently their corresponding bodily alterations. The synergy of both treatments has always benefitted the patients. I, too, as your patient, have been well treated, with great professionalism, care, and dedication. Finally, I wish you the best with your book, which will be much appreciated by our colleagues and patients.*

— *DR. LUIS BRIL ROSEMBERG*, MEDICAL DOCTOR AND SURGEON. SPECIALIST IN ESTHETIC MEDICINE AT THE MADRID COMPLUTENSE UNIVERSITY. PLASTIC, RECONSTRUCTIVE, AND ESTHETIC SURGERY.

# 9

# Colonic Hydrotherapy –
# The Body's Roadworthiness Test

As we have learnt in previous chapters, the intestinal microflora in your gut is a key player in health. If the intestinal ecology of the gut is not in balance, and the diet inadequate, then over time the colon begins to show irritation at the level of the mucosa and hard, acidic, and rotten deposits begin to stick to the walls of the intestine.

Even if evacuation is completely normal, sticky toxic residues stay stuck to the folds of the intestine. They progressively accumulate and end up "fouling" the colon, forming a crust. The dirt can come to cover many parts of the large intestine with these hardened plaques and impede its functioning. This, in turn, leads to imbalanced microflora and reduces the local defenses, creating a vicious cycle.

This toxic process can be compared with the pipework of your house when there is an accumulation of lime. If you turn on a tap when the pipes are partially blocked by the lime, the water comes out but with less force and is of poorer quality; it can even can become undrinkable. When this happens, you wouldn't hesitate to call a plumber to come and check the system as soon as possible, and you would carry out some preventive work to avoid future problems, such as fitting a filter. Agreed?

The same happens with our "pipes." We expel the residue, but each time in lesser quantities and without tackling the buildup on the walls. The quality of the feces gets worse, converting more into acid and bad smells and irritating the anus, making it itchy and encouraging the formation of hemorrhoids and anal fissures.

General clinical medical practice confirms that no patient is free of intestinal disorders. As we have seen, across the world millions of people suffer from mild to chronic irritable bowel syndrome, and millions more suffer with severe constipation. A number of people have a high probability of developing cancer of the colon during their lives.

Pathologists who perform autopsies and study the tissues of cadavers report that 60–70 percent of the colons they examine contain fecal material as hard as stone and decades old. According to the World Health Organization, 80 percent of cancers and metabolic illnesses can be prevented through an adequate diet that leads to a healthy digestion. That's 80 percent! Don't you want to sign up?

As it is not always easy to modify your eating habits, avoid stress, or exercise regularly, it can be of great help to know about natural measures and techniques that are effective for improving intestinal elimination.

One such method, colonic hydrotherapy, is available to anyone who wants to improve his vitality and health. Its offers several beneficial effects, and results are seen quickly. These include an immediate sensation of lightness and well-being, weight loss, better mental functioning, and a noticeable improvement in physiological functions. A properly functioning gut is a basis for good health.

Some people, however, find the idea of cleaning out their intestines a little off-putting. To run water through the colon is no more risky than rinsing out your mouth or gargling. The colon is not sterile, and cleansing the intestine doesn't harm the intestinal flora—rather, it noticeably improves it.

Many hospitals in various countries of the world cleanse the intestines of a patient before a colonoscopy or before abdominal surgery, even in serious cases.

## History of Internal Cleansing

As mentioned earlier, for thousands of years human have tried to improve their health by cleaning their insides. The antecedents of colonic hydrotherapy can be seen in the intestinal cleansings mentioned in Sumerian, Chinese, Hindu, Greek, and Roman texts, although they were recorded in most detail in the papyruses of ancient Egypt. As we have noted, in AD 77, the Roman philosopher, historian, and naturalist Pliny the Elder reported on the legend of the ibis, which showed man how to purge his intestine. After having an abundant meal of fish, this bird felt overloaded. With its beak it sucked up water from the sea and introducing it into its anus, afterward expelling it and feeling better.

In the 19th century, colonic hydrotherapy was used and promoted in the United States by Dr. John Harvey Kellogg, famous for the invention of breakfast cereals. Kellogg was a revolutionary doctor who used holistic methods in medicine, placing particular importance on nutrition, physical exercise, and making extensive therapeutic use of enemas. He was a committed vegetarian and practiced colonic hydrotherapy himself throughout his life. In his articles for *The Journal of the American Medical Association* (JAMA), he recommended colonic hydrotherapy for almost all ailments and proved its effect in clinical cases. Using colonic hydrotherapy, he managed to stabilize and improve the health of numerous patients with systemic illnesses. Despite living in difficult times, he lived to the ripe old age of 92, enjoying good health and remaining lucid until the end of his life. He died in 1943.

Intestinal cleansing continued to be used by American doctors and was in fashion until the 1970s. There was even a "Colonic Row" in Beverley Hills, home of the rich and privileged of California. There are many archives from this period on the therapeutic use of colonic hydrotherapy in Europe, too, in the imperial spas of Germany, Austria, France, and Switzerland. Since the 1970s, however, intestinal hygiene has been increasingly neglected in favor of the treatment of symptoms with chemical medications. All systems of traditional and natural medicine, however, have always been in favor of this treatment.

The most important people in the development of colonic hydrotherapy in the 20th century include doctors Kellogg, B. Jensen, P. Carton, Lagroua, Bertholet, C. Vasey, V. Irons, and Kousmine.

## Colon Hydrotherapy Today

The value of natural therapies and preventive techniques is increasingly recognized, and there has especially been an increase in the use of colonic hydrotherapy. The modern patient is better informed and knows more about natural methods and their efficacy in improving quality of life. Colonic hydrotherapy has resumed its therapeutic place and is available in many hospitals and well-being clinics around the world. In addition, colonic hydrotherapy is the focus of interest from biological medicine, as a tool for cellular detoxification and the prevention of aging.

The United States is the world leader in holistic medicine, including colonic hydrotherapy. In Europe, the use of colonic hydrotherapy is well developed in Britain, Germany, and Switzerland, as well as in the mineral water spas of the Czech Republic and Hungary. In Germany and Switzerland, intestinal cleaning is as common as dental work or skincare. Many people are totally receptive to the idea of intestinal cleaning and the knowledge that by using this method they can help prevent colon cancer is enough to persuade them to have an annual maintenance colonic. German sausages and beer may be habits that are difficult to break, but at least an annual digestive "vehicle" inspection offers some compensation.

In the United Kingdom, colonic hydrotherapy is offered at almost all important clinics practicing alternative medicine. One of the London clinics patronized by Prince Charles, for example, has several colonic hydrotherapy rooms. To the British, a classical education and good manners are completely compatible with keeping their digestive systems tidy through assisted cleaning. In fact, in Britain, colonic hydrotherapy is covered by some insurance companies.

In several places in Europe colonic hydrotherapy is integrated into medical centers for the treatment of digestive disorders. Using colonic hydrotherapy, any patient can be prepared for a colonoscopy in an hour, or for surgery on the digestive tract, without having to wait or suffer preparations using laxatives, as happens in the majority of hospitals.

· · · · · · · ·

In the Czech Republic, which was for a long time influenced by Germany and Austria, hydrotherapy has deep roots. It is worth mentioning a small and famous city called Karlovy Vary, which is situated on the border with Germany, 130 km (80 miles) from the city of Prague. It is also called Karlsbad (the spa town of the Emperor Charles). The city is hidden in a valley protected by mountains and has an exclusive climate.

Its famed spa draws on 12 types of natural thermal water, which are differentiated by their temperature, mineral composition, and therapeutic properties. Most of them are used for the treatment of digestive disorders. With such a range of thermal waters there are many therapeutic possibilities for all types of digestive and metabolic illnesses. The city has been famous since the 14th century because of its many stories of cures, and its health-giving waters have made it a privileged place of treatment for noble and royal families.

Remarkably, the spa facilities and promenades of the old part of Karlovy Vary still maintain their imperial air and style from centuries past. When you arrive there is nothing else to do but relax, stroll, rest, take the waters, and regenerate your digestive tract mucosa (unless you decide to spend the night indulging yourself drinking Czech beers, but I don't recommend this).

Most spas have their colonic hydrotherapy departments. These are the only places where intestinal irrigation is carried out directly using thermal waters because the pipes of these centers are directly connected to mineral springs.

In developed countries, in recent years, there has been increasing interest in colonic hydrotherapy, both among patients and among medical doctors and doctors of naturopathic medicine. It is now available in clinics in many cities. Personal treatment, prices, the quality of advice given, and the level of monitoring can, of course, vary greatly from clinic to clinic.

## The Process of Colonic Hydrotherapy

What exactly is colonic hydrotherapy? Is it a large-scale enema performed in a sophisticated manner, or is there something deeper to it? In reality it is much more complex.

A colonic hydrotherapy session consists of the gentle introduction of previously filtered and purified water into the colon via the rectum in a safe and systematic way. Depending on therapeutic requirements, the colon may be irrigated with water enriched with ozone, individualized preparations of medicinal plants, or cocktails of prebiotics. All this helps the treatment and localized healing of the mucosa. During the session, it is beneficial to carry out multiple fillings and emptyings, to practice breathing techniques, and to apply gentle abdominal massage.

Modern colonic hydrotherapy equipment enables a precise control and adjustment of the different elements used in treatment. It produces a complete and effective cleaning of the large intestine with a high level of safety.

The automatic, instantaneous system of filling and emptying helps to dissolve all the deposits stuck firmly in the colon. During a colonic hydrotherapy treatment, the discharge of fecal residue passes through a transparent, illuminated tube that allows the specialist operative to make observations and receive information useful for diagnosis. During the procedure, a cannula (a tube like a catheter) is used. This is connected to two circuits of tubes, permitting the entry of pure water and the independent exit of water loaded with residues. The treatment is completely closed to external contamination because of the use of disposable materials. After every session, the equipment is automatically disinfected. A colonic hydrotherapy treatment takes 35–45 minutes and uses 20–30 liters (35–50 pints) of cleansing water in total.

In order to achieve a complete and effective deep therapeutic cleaning, three treatments are recommended, at intervals determined by the doctor reviewing the initial state of the digestive system. The first session will clean out residual material that has been impacted for a long time, relieve flatulence, and sometimes take away several kilos of weight; the second and third sessions are the ones where a deep and complete cleansing of the colon is achieved, effective over the long term.

Colonic hydrotherapy is completely hygienic, painless, without odor, and is not in any way disagreeable. You may, however, experience some discomfort as a result of constipation, spasticity of the colon, excessive flatulence, and the sensation of soft pressure when the water fills the colon—along with a great sense of relief with each discharge. During the session, the patient can communicate with the practitioner carrying out the treatment in any moment, and he or she can comment on the sensations felt. After the session, the patient receives dietary advice and suggestions for natural substances to take, such as probiotics, then goes back to normal life.

When you undergo a session of colonic hydrotherapy you are dressed in a gown or apron and lie on a bed covered with a sheet. When the rectal examination is carried out and the cannula is introduced, you will be asked to lie in the fetal position. When preparing you for treatment, the nurse-hydrotherapist will cover your private parts, and these will not be visible or exposed to external contact.

As some people don't know what is involved and how colonic hydrotherapy is carried out, which is normal, they try to adopt an elbows-to-knees posture with their backsides raised vertically like a flag, or else they expect to see something similar to a gynecological chair. A very few people who have an exaggerated, pathological sense of shame, try to hide themselves, covering their heads with a pillow and sending out the clear message, "I am not me and I'm not here," or else they behave as if the ugly stuff that comes out of them has nothing do with their bodies. The majority of people accept the procedure once they are connected to the machine, and they quickly get comfortable (because the staff usually treat them so well). They want to know everything that is happening and to know about everything that comes out of them, behaving like fascinated children when they discover its contents and abundance. In general, everyone has a good experience. It is a challenge and also a way of learning about yourself. To have a session of colonic hydrotherapy guarantees you a benefit. Whether you suffer or enjoy the process, you will lose a few kilos (pounds) of residues and toxins from your body.

## A Roadworthiness Test for the Body

Your body is like a vehicle that you drive around in, which accommodates the mind and consciousness. We are full of ideas, thoughts, dreams, and ambitions, but for us to make any of these things come true we must keep our means of transport well maintained and functioning. This doesn't happen by itself; we have to participate. We have to give our bodies a checkup and service every now and then. In my clinic, we offer a program we call "Fine Tuning the Digestive System." At the very least, I urge you to carry out an inspection of your "vehicle," so that afterward you can take the other steps toward good health. Life changes are not accomplished overnight.

The authorities oblige us to keep our cars in perfect condition for reasons of road safety, and if you ignore the appropriate vehicle inspection of roadworthiness you get a fine. Don't you dare protest; it's a very clear rule: your car has to be safe to prevent accidents and harm to others. I would love one day for the health system and society to set similar rules for the inspection of our bodies, obliging us to give them the minimum of care necessary to maintain their mental and physical health, and to prevent the accidents and damage that can occur when we are on the highway of life.

It is not my intention to suggest that everyone should have colonic hydrotherapy sessions. I am merely talking about reeducating people about digestion and that they should control their weight, diet, level of physical activity, quality of rest, and how they care for their digestive and general health. What are the immediate short-term benefits associated with colonic hydrotherapy?

- **The volume of the colon**—and of the gut in general—is reduced by eliminating the majority or the totality of the intestinal contents.
- **A reduction in pressure** on the neighboring organs and the diaphragm takes place, which leads to relaxation and improved breathing. There is a sense of relief and agreeable emptiness and well-being inside your belly.

- **The reduction of the pressure inside the abdomen favors the venolym-pathic circulation from the legs and the hemorrhoidal area** and this noticeably improves symptoms related to the retention of liquids and of venolymphatic insufficiency. It improves and helps control the effects of painful and abundant menstruation and of premenstrual syndrome.
- **Decongestion and decompression** of the lumbar and sacral areas of the spinal column (the accumulation of gas and of feces in the guts can press from within and causes blockages). This improves the functioning of the articulations of the hip sockets and notably relieves lumbar and sciatic pain.
- **Healing and renewal.** Colonic hydrotherapy has a calming and anti-inflammatory effect on the intestine walls, which soothes an irritable colon and constipation. Once cleaned of the buildup of toxic elements and old mucus, and aided by an adequate diet, the intestinal epithelium is capable of regrowing itself in about five days, generating a new lubricating mucus that favors the balance of microflora in the colon.
- **Detoxification.** This benefits all the body's systems, but the most immediate effects are improvement in the psychoemotional state, including better mental functioning and reductions in insomnia, depression, anxiety, and migraines; improvements in atopic dermatitis, eczema, psoriasis, and acne; retention of interstitial fluids in the connective tissue is also noticed.

And long-term effects?

- Stimulation of the immune system
- Corrected digestion, as a result of better absorption and more complete passage of nutrients and substances into the bloodstream
- Improved memory and functioning of the central nervous system
- Vitality of the intestinal mucosa with the formation of a balanced microflora
- Regular motility in the large intestine
- Positive changes to metabolism

## Conditions Suitable for Colonic Hydrotherapy

Colonic hydrotherapy is recommended for all adults as a preventive measure to maintain health and well-being. It is most commonly recommended for the following conditions (previously assessed by a doctor):

- Constipation
- Chronic diarrhea

- Weakness or flaccidity of the colon
- Abundance of gas and flatulence
- Irritable colon
- Obesity and excess weight
- Chronic inflammatory illnesses
- Metabolic illnesses
- Skin problems
- Allergies, in general
- Menstrual problems
- Stress, insomnia, anxiety
- Circulatory problems—slow flow and return in the veins and lymph vessels, leading to water retention and swelling
- Prevention of aging
- Preparation for carrying out a colonoscopy and certain surgical procedures.

## Contraindications for Colonic Hydrotherapy

The following conditions require doctor's approval before undertaking colonic hydrotherapy treatment:

- Surgery carried out within the previous six months
- Decompensated ulcerative colitis
- Cancer of the colon
- Acute or serious cardiovascular illnesses
- Serious anemia
- Inguinal hernia
- Aortic aneurism
- Neurological illnesses
- Pregnancy.

## Colonic Hydrotherapy and Chronic Disease

Colonic hydrotherapy is an important tool for treating patients with chronic conditions, as it can be used in cases where the patient is, or has been, using pharmaceutical medications for a prolonged period of time. Colonic hydrotherapy improves the absorption of medications, as well as essential nutrients in the body. Routine colonic hydrotherapy treatments led to a significant reduction in the dosages of medications required and length of treatment. It also helps boost the production of immune cells by the intestinal mucosa, as well as promotes adequate hydration and detoxification in the body after it has been subjected to aggressive treatment protocols. Cancer patients suffer many side effects from radiotherapy and chemotherapy, which cause multiple gastrointestinal alterations. These treatments interfere with a patient's quality of life and affect their psychological state. Various natural methods, among them colonic hydrotherapy, help improve the condition of these patients, but it is essential that medical professionals coordinate care of such patients before treatments take place.

* * * * * * * *

Patient B., 53 years old. In 2010, I underwent surgery for breast cancer and was subsequently given a treatment based on tamoxifen. Although I have always had a lazy intestine, in the last 15 years I have solved the problem by following an appropriate diet. However, when I began chemotherapy, my intestine stopped functioning and, of course, I had no intention of taking laxatives because I knew the undesirable consequences of using them. Aware of the poor functioning of such an important organ, I was very anxious because I didn't know what to do to solve this problem. So I decided to try colonic hydrotherapy treatment in Dr. Irina Matveikova's Clinic of Digestive Health. I remember with gratitude the care and delicacy with which the work was carried out by her assistant, María, who performs the colonic hydrotherapy treatments in the clinic under the supervision of the doctor.

From the first colonic hydrotherapy session I noticed a spectacular change in my intestine, which went from being totally blocked to problem-free daily functioning. With much care – given that after the postsurgical radiotherapy I had been diagnosed with pneumonitis – Dr. Irina treated me step by step, first deeply cleaning my colon and supplying the necessary nutrients for it to heal. This was an important advance towards my recovery, and I noticed immediate results. From the outset, the doctor recommended a treatment to prepare for detoxification of the liver, and this was another important and significant step in improving my intestinal transit, followed thereafter by a detoxification treatment of the kidneys.

My digestive system is functioning pretty well now, although it is also true that while I am receiving chemotherapy I will need to have periodic sessions of colonic hydrotherapy to keep my colon functioning. The peace of mind brought by a treatment in which the doctor is interested not only in my progress but also in my diet is something I appreciate greatly. I feel that I have taken a giant step forward in my health, in general, including my state of mind. I sincerely believe that a healthy body, free of impurities, has an impact not only on the psychic level but also on the emotional level and, of course, on the spiritual level.

It is very simple and clear: by having your colon cared for, cleaned out, and its natural ecology restored, you stay in control of your digestive health and much more—reason enough to overcome inertia, laziness, shyness, and any unnecessary shame and "sacrifice" your backside to the treatment.

Colonic hydrotherapy is not a cure, nor is it is a solution for all that ails you. But it is no small thing to detoxify and reduce inflammation in such an enormous intestinal area and restore its ecological balance so that it can adequately absorb nutrients and stay on top of the billions of bacterial inhabitants that live there. Colonic hydrotherapy cuts down on the work load of trying to accomplish all this entirely on your own. It supports your liver and your body's entire detoxification system, so that they can use their energy to deal with more important tasks.

I hope that I have convinced you that ridding yourself of the toxic, smelly waste in your "temple" is a good habit to incorporate into your life.

Let me now share some distant memories of a teaching doctor, a German naturopath, who was committed to his profession and passionate about it (he was elderly but healthy and with the energy and vitality of a young man). Sometimes he gave his patients a "very special demonstration" of the dirt inside them, and he did it in the following way.

What you try to ignore a gut that is full of feces for many days—because you have forgotten, are tired of fighting with your innards, don't have time, or don't know what more you can do—you are taking this totalitarian decision without consulting your body. The digestive, lymphatic, and immune systems don't have a vote or any rights to interfere or protest, so you leave them with an internal "environmental disaster," one your body has to "swallow." Okay, you say, nothing's wrong. You take your time, continue with your life. But to be fair and democratic and to understand your "subordinates," you need to take responsibility for your acts and share the environment with them.

When this crazy old man saw patients with constipation (those who weren't very clear about what was happening to them, or the damage they were doing to their bodies, and came to ask him about other matters), he would place on the desk, near the patient, a bowl full of feces, the quantity in proportion to the size of the patient and the duration of his intestinal blockage. If the patient was a large man or woman with 4–5 days of backlog, the bowl would be very big and would be filled with a couple of kilos of foul-smelling fecal matter.

As you can imagine, his patients were very surprised. Then, in typical phlegmatic German fashion, the doctor would tell them that there was nothing wrong, that he was showing them simply what they had chosen to keep in their bodies, the essence of their gut on that day—and they should imagine that massive excrement growing in their bodies daily. The doctor continued with his demonstration until he got the patient's full awareness. For him, it was very simple: Are you going to clean out your insides? Or do you want to take this bowl home with you?

This anecdote may seem brutal, but the truth is that the doctor had a good reputation. In the end, people like to be told things clearly.

The surprising success of the television series *House* is due to the fact that even though the protagonist has a brusque, rude character and a horrible attitude toward everyone, in the end he is brilliant and saves lives. It seems that, on occasion, people like to be repulsed. We could say that it is necessary to see and talk about unpleasant things in order to wake up.

I promise that in our clinic we don't do anything as brutal and rude as this. Modern colonic hydrotherapy avoids any contact with your residues, the process of cleansing is sterile, and the nurses treat patients with care. I well know that it takes a lot for a new patient to make the decision to come in for treatment, and because of this I have maximum respect for his intimacy.

Colonic hydrotherapy is a therapeutic tool. We talk about it with the patient, examine him and assess his health, and together we plan some changes and solutions. After treatment, we keep in touch with him and send out reminders to come in for regular checkups. The clinical relationship begins with colonic cleansing and never ends. I always say to new patients, "Welcome to the club," because no one disappears forever. In general, they don't usually call when they feel well, but some do.

I have a patient, P., who has *Crohn's disease* (chronic inflammation of part of the colon leading to the formation of deep ulcers and episodes of bleeding). Treating her has required a good deal of care. It has not been easy, because it means paying a lot of attention to the treatment of intestines that are very inflamed, a big responsibility. We have now spent three years in the maintenance phase and seen a clear remission in her illness. P. feels well—really well—and lives just like a normal person, without limitations or fears.

Each time she calls me my heart jumps in case she is doing so because she has had an acute outbreak or has begun to bleed. But P. calls only to tell me that she is well, and nothing else, or to ask me if she has to come in for a checkup. I want to share her testimony with you:

• • • • • • • • •

I am 54 years old. When I was 43, I was diagnosed with inflammatory bowel disease. It is a chronic illness, of uncertain origin, which comes in bursts and has periods of remission. It manifests as ulcers in the colon and abdominal pain, diarrhea with blood in the stools, sometimes fever, and anemia, and a general sensation of tiredness and weakness making it hard to live a normal life.

From the beginning, I have followed conventional medical treatment for the disease, which consists of daily medication and the use of corticosteroids during the illness's active phases. At first the treatment seemed effective. I had a period of inactivity of approximately one year, when there was a complete remission of symptoms. After that, though, for no apparent reason, there were fresh, more prolonged attacks, with more acute symptoms and increasingly longer periods of inactivity.

Three years ago, I underwent my first colonic hydrotherapy treatment, which consisted of a rigorous diet that included many natural supplements and several cycles of gentle intestinal irrigation enriched with the doctor's personal herbal preparations and ozone. This produced a noticeable effect almost immediately. Since then, my intestinal function has practically gone back to normal. My abdominal pains have disappeared, I no longer have blood in my stools, and I have gone back to enjoying a life full of energy, a varied diet, and am able to travel. My doctor and I stay in touch, and I am aware that in spite of feeling well, we cannot completely stop pharmaceutical treatment of the ulcerative colitis prescribed by my gastroenterologist. However, working together my medical team has managed to halve the dosages of my medications, and for years now I have not used anti-inflammatory suppositories nor do I need corticosteroids.

In all this time there has only been one small outbreak, of short duration, and with light symptoms, which seems to have been caused by a viral infection.

## Emotional Effects of Colonic Hydrotherapy

In addition to internal cleansing, colonic hydrotherapy mobilizes and detoxifies the digestive system and encourages emotional and energetic movement. According to traditional Chinese medicine, negative energy flows through the intestinal tract in order to leave the body, so it must always be kept clean and open. The meridian that corresponds with the intestine is associated with negative thoughts, fear, and anger. At the same time, the intestine is where traumas, frustrations, hidden memories, fears, and even phobias can hide. When you "take the lid off," you let these things flow and clean them out with purified water; it is like a performing a ritual—deep and emotional.

The trust that the patient places in you, in complete confidentiality, allows energy to move in the *hara*, the navel *chakra*, the *energetic canal* or *meridian*—names associated with various cultures, essentially those of Asian origin. During the therapy, many patients open their minds and hearts and begin to talk about very personal things. It seems as if they are drowning under waves of emotions that haven't been expressed, and which they don't want to keep inside them any more. By allowing water to flow through their innards beyond their control, it is as if they let their emotions and energies flow at the same time, without holding back.

This doesn't happen to everyone, of course—least of all during the initial treatment. During that first session of colonic hydrotherapy, the patient is still not familiar with the situation and the sensations. During the treatment he receives a lot of new information, and some people find this a bit overwhelming at the beginning. In subsequent sessions, however, when they feel more confident and understand what the procedure consists of, their psychoemotional state changes greatly.

As energy moves in your "second brain" during deep purification, your soul can suddenly feel bare and vulnerable, with overflowing thoughts and emotions. It is very supportive in these moments to have someone—the doctor and/or therapist—listen to you. For this reason, at the clinic we choose our therapists with great care and ask that they be fully trained in psychotherapy and/or energetic therapies. The patient simultaneously experiences a tremendous sense of relief and feels very confused and exposed, but a connection between doctor and patient has been created, which is necessary for there to be a good rapport between them.

I remember one patient—a well-known actress who always seems luminous, happy, and smiling. In a particular moment, she broke down in tears during a session of colonic hydrotherapy and began to talk about the recent death of her father, drowning in her sense of guilt. In another case, a famous theater actor began to talk about the hatred he felt toward his sister. Many people return to the memories of infancy and their personal relationships and share their frustrations.

I am not the only one who observes this type of reaction. There are publications in the United States on this subject. For example, Dr. R. Anderson of San Francisco has been working for more than half a century in the area of bodily detoxification and colonic hydrotherapy. He writes in his book that his patients undergo tremendous psychological and emotional releases as their colons are purified. He discusses what is known as "cellular memory." The theory is that every strong emotion we have leaves an energetic imprint in the body, meaning simply that such emotions are so concentrated and have such an impact on us, they leave an electromagnetic impression and stay recorded in our biological tissues. Our bodies store facts and memories much like we do with digital media; in this case, what we call cellular memory is a memory deposit in our intestinal mucosa.

We have already talked about how we are normally entirely renewable. Our bodies automatically reline our digestive tracts, discard cells, and build new ones and update our tissues little by little, replacing old building blocks with new ones. Everything is constantly renewing. But when the large intestine is saturated with mucus and old toxic residues, the process of cellular renewal and the shedding of dead epithelial cells slows down, and can even come to a halt.

The accumulated mucus and cells in the digestive tract are like an old library filled with old books that are never read. When you begin the process of purification, this layer of dirt is swept away, and the words in those old books begin to be heard, bringing back memories that have been stored and perhaps almost forgotten. This is what is suddenly stirred up in the patient. It is as if he is able to listen again to his emotions and relive them, but in a different way, learning from them. According to Dr. Anderson, it is a moving process, and it is important to guide the patient professionally. Colonic hydrotherapy can discharge not only old residues but also the heaviness of emotions that haven't been resolved.

I am perhaps more conservative. I withhold judgment and have no comment on such an *avant-garde*—or perhaps old—philosophical theory, although it seems to me an interesting metaphorical concept. What I have no doubt about, however—and in this, I agree completely with Dr. Anderson—is that during colonic hydrotherapy sessions, patients are moved emotionally as well as physically, and this helps them a lot in the process of purification.

Before publication of this book in Spain, my publisher asked me to back up what I have to say with testimonials from famous people, that is to say references from those of my patients who are well known or important. The theory is that this will give me credibility with my readers and interest the media, given that people love to know a bit about the private life of celebrities. Not to indulge in false modesty, but I do indeed have many famous patients who are involved in the arts in Spain, as well as several VIPs and experts in their field. These people come into my consulting room, and you might think that their famous names alone would be enough to warrant special treatment. But because I am a foreigner, don't know many people, and am not up to date with the celebrity gossip magazines, I instead treat them as mere mortals out of simple ignorance. I can confirm that, despite everything, such people like to be normal, natural, and sincere, without being given special treatment.

Let me offer one anecdote. Around three years ago, a glamorous star of the gossip magazines called me on my mobile phone (in person!), giving me her name and leaving a long pause so that I could take in to whom I was speaking. That day, however, I was minus my assistant and overloaded with consultations and therapies, so I was not able to give her my full attention; instead, I asked her to call back later. She tried to contact me several times that day, and finally, the diva started shouting that she was famous and important and did not have time to wait and that I should give her an appointment. It was such an impressive shout that even the patient I was with could hear it! She began to motion to me that I needed to attend to somebody so famous immediately. So I did. Later I was told who she was, and finally I had the pleasure of knowing and treating her. We still have a friendly relationship today, and I'm glad that I have been able to help with her digestive health.

While I have shared the testimonials of several well-known patients who were willing to discuss my work, I cannot share with you the names and stories of those celebrities who come to me in confidence, as these are very intimate and personal. I prefer to maintain a zone of privacy for these celebrities and not force them to share their experiences with the press and the public, in general. I appeal to your intuitive sensibilities to enjoy my book and look for what is positive in it without me having to give attention-grabbing endorsements. And right now, I thank you for that.

*My problems with diet began when, as my career took off, I was put into this whirlwind of work and all my eating habits changed: days of lunches with clients and colleagues ran into other days when the need to finish some project didn't leave me time to eat. To this was added the fact that, when I got home from work at night, dinner became my most peaceful moment, and I released my stress by devouring everything that was in the fridge.*

*Right now, I am in the process of controling all this. I try to live with the stress, without jeopardizing my present or future private life by being overweight. Dr. Irina has helped me—above all, when it comes to motivation—to make a change in my life through dietary reeducation and also refocusing my life, enabling me to understand that my day-to-day life must change, and with it my dietary habits.*

*Healthy eating is an important subject today, and requires study of each person's particular situation and unique health problems in order to tailor a diet designed to treat the individual. This is why I am grateful to the author, who has looked into my problem not only from the point of view of diet but also of my lifestyle.*

— *JOSE ANTONIO HERNANDEZ MARTIN, SENIOR MANAGER HEALTHCARE AND LIFE SCIENCE ADVISORY, BUSINESS PERFORMANCE SERVICES, KPMG CONSULTANTS*

# 10

# Intestinal Microflora – Myths and Truths

The media gives us constant messages about the importance of maintaining the defenses in our intestines, insisting that we have to eat and drink various yogurts of different brands every day. This kind of advertising seems to me useful for a basic public education on the care of our intestinal ecology, even if the advisers' promises, inevitably made for commercial reasons, may be exaggerated.

Many people are not clear about the meaning of the term *intestinal microflora*—and understand words such as *probiotics* and *prebiotics* even less. Nevertheless, they are highly influenced by what they hear on television and think: "If I drink this brand of yogurt every day, I will boost my immunological defences, control my cholesterol, and possibly solve my problems of constipation." The intention is good, and certainly, it is good for a person who is healthy and balanced to eat these products daily; however, if tummy upsets and digestive problems persist, these over-the-counter measures are insufficient and do not solve the problem. In my consulting room I often hear the following:

- If I am consuming a yogurt drink every day, which the advertisers claim will increase my immune defenses, why do I have colds so often? This winter is killing me!
- When my son drank a yogurt drink advertised to boost the body's defenses, he got much better.
- Why should I take pills for cholesterol? I will just consume a yogurt drink that the advertisements say will help reduce my cholesterol.
- I eat two or three pots of yogurts a day, and I am still constipated!
- My GP has told me that I have high cholesterol and has prescribed a yogurt drink that decreases blood cholesterol levels.
- I know I have osteoporosis, but I consume a yogurt drink with extra calcium to strengthen my bones. I don't want to take another form of calcium.
- I know that yogurt is good, but it gives me heartburn. I feel bad. I don't know what to do.

- Milk fortified with calcium and Omega 3 fatty acids protects my heart. I don't need anything else.

Here we can see a common mistake. *Functional foods* (foods that have added active ingredients to provide more nutrients), such as yogurts and other fermented dairy (or vegetable) products, do form part of a balanced and healthy nutritional intake. Consumed regularly, they help keep us healthy and prevent problems with intestinal ecology; however, they do not provide a cure in themselves, and they are not a substitute for medical care as a first measure in treating a problem. We have to recover and strengthen our internal bacterial equilibrium first, then maintain it with functional foods afterwards.

## What Do We Mean by Intestinal Microflora?

We use the term "intestinal microflora" to refer to our own personal zoology, a universe of diverse bacteria, viruses, fungi, yeasts, and parasites that live in our intestines. It is normal for the intestinal tract to be filled with bacteria, but some less friendly strains of bacteria can invade our intestines and take up residence there.

The intestinal microflora of an adult includes more than 400 strains of bacteria and literally hundreds of millions of individual bacteria. Each bacterium is a one-celled organism; together this potent biomass generates an intense metabolic activity in the colon and strongly influences the physiology of the host. They are so numerous, in fact, they make up 40–50 percent of the weight of the feces.

Your feces are an accumulation of bacteria. Those that are expelled by the body's "presiding authority" in the gut are those bacteria that have not been able to justify their prolonged presence there and have not found a niche where they can take up residence.

Our bodies are assemblies of billions of cells, but the total number of one-celled bacteria accommodated in our colon is 10 times higher and more concentrated than in the rest of our body. It is a powerful melting pot of cultures—numerous, important, and impossible to ignore.

## A Universe in Your Gut

We are humans on Planet Earth. In comparison with the size of the universe, our solar system, our "blue ball," even, we are less than ants: relatively speaking, we human beings are like the tiny one-celled bacteria that live inside the larger universe of our bodies.

From the vantage point of space, we humans are unimportant, invisible. The laws of the universe continue to unfold, no matter what. In any moment, we could destroy ourselves or be destroyed. We could be transformed into space dust from the impact of a meteorite colliding with the earth, or be irradiated by the sun. We might be invaded by extraterrestials—or come to face the final apocalypse.

We are not passive beings, though, even if we look small and miserable when viewed from another planet. Little by little, drop by drop, we influence our own universe. We send spaceships and observation stations into space. We destroy the ozone layer and contaminate the earth. Our actions provoke epidemics and global warming, and we suffer the ensuing floods and droughts. If Earth is not well; if it is in upheaval; if its own ecology is out of balance; if its burgeoning population of microscopic inhabitants is damaging its health—all this influences the universe in some way.

Where am I going with this? It seems to me that this way of looking at universal processes could be useful to the reader in understanding the "universe" of our intestinal microflora.

We carry within our bodies the "universes" inhabited by multiple bacteria. We don't, however, give them much importance and they don't "mean anything" to us in the context of our development and our daily problems. We could destroy them in an instant with antibiotics, eliminate them with severe diarrhea, and harm them with drugs and toxins. In short, each of us is a universe governed by laws and decisions that are frequently fatal for bacteria!

Nevertheless, the numerous inhabitants of our colons, the "intestinal microflora," know very well how to influence their "planet." They may act all "Greenpeace" and "environmentalist," delivering vitamins and nutrients, boosting our defenses, improving our digestion and our total health. Or they may be be unconscious and ignorant and provoke "wars" and even be dominated by aggressive invaders, provoking a high level of contamination in the gut through gas and toxins. In this way, they may seriously damage their host: us.

They are very similar to us, aren't they? They are just a different size. Every bacterium has to eat and excrete, compete for food, struggle for its niche (house), and is obliged to comply with the rules of living together.

A balanced intestinal microflora (a healthy internal ecology) is a mass of predominantly "good," almost vegetarian bacteria that are highly aware of their environment. These bacteria maintain friendly and very diplomatic relations with our intestinal mucosa. It is a highly holistic and intelligent ecosystem, with many interrelationships, not only with other bacteria but also with the rest of the body. Among the many benefits of a healthy intestinal microflora, the most important is to nourish the *enterocytes* (the cells of the intestine) and contribute to a local immunological response for the defense of the human body.

An unbalanced intestinal microflora (*dysbiosis*) is a growth of "bad" bacteria that attack each other and the cells of the colon, producing great irritation and generating a process of local inflammation. These strains are carnivorous—they prefer proteins—and by-products of their disorganized lives are very toxic and damaging to the host: they provoke putrefaction in protein residues and mutations in the cells of the colon.

Dysbiosis can also be caused by fungal strains, such as *candida albicans*, and yeasts—"beasts" that love sweets, and carbohydrates in general, which they "devour." They immediately ferment sugars and thereby generate gas in industrial quantities.

In extreme disequilibrium, the intestinal microflora can transform itself into an aggressive, invader biomass that causes the development of digestive illnesses, the growth and development of polyps, cancer of the colon, and toxicity in the body in general.

### How the Intestinal Microflora is Formed

Everything that grows in our gut has entered through the mouth since the day we were born. The normal development of the intestinal microflora during infancy can be divided into four very important phases that have to be controlled and corrected at the time:

- The initial acquisition of microorganisms at the moment of birth
- The period of breastfeeding
- The beginning of complementary food
- The beginning of an adult diet

Intestinal microflora do not live everywhere in the digestive tract. In a healthy stomach, for example, there are almost no bacteria present because of the highly acidic environment (pH1). A very limited quantity of microorganisms manage to survive after coming into contact with the stomach juices, which is extremely acidic, and go on to the next part of the intestinal tract, the duodenum. The environment in the duodenum is more agreeable to bacteria, due to its neutral pH (around 7), but bacteria do not have much time to relax and reproduce there because they are rapidly attacked by the bile and the pancreatic juices.

Despite permanent attacks by enzymes, there are certain strains of microbes that are more resistant and manage to survive in the small intestine and reach the colon; however, there are few of them, and this process of advancing through hostile environments means that they cannot multiply or gain the strength necessary to influence their immediate environment.

In order to maintain adequate proportions of bacteria in the colon, it has to receive "special divisions" of "good" bacteria that are selected and trained to resist extreme situations, with the "mission" of arriving at their final destination and surviving—at least some of them. They have to do this continually, and in rein forced groups. These special divisions of friendly bacteria are called *probiotics*, and their mission is to enter the colon in therapeutic doses (special supplements). A probiotic literally means "messenger that promotes life." We are talking about a community of living beings (they contain strains of live bacteria) that may or may not die on the journey.

Imagine now that yogurt or fermented milk drink that promises to benefit your health. What probability is there, do you think, of this inoffensive "civilian worker" arriving safe and whole in your colon? Yogurt is a useful probiotic but does not contain levels of friendly bacteria in the necessary therapeutic concentrations. Instead, the doses are merely preventive, designed to maintain the equilibrium already achieved. Do you understand the difference?

## Bacteria and Their "Social Classes"

We are now going to complicate the subject a little. The intelligent "microbe state" that we have in our innards has its own rules and social divisions. They include:

- **DOMINANT BACTERIA:** These are families of permanent residents who have their own rights and social privileges and their own territories— "estates"—that correspond to sections or portions of our intestinal mucosa. These bacteria are stuck intimately to our cells by means of a dense layer of mucus that we ourselves produce, and that serves as a *niche*, or a place of containment, for this microbial colony.

    This layer of mucus is made up of an intelligent gel formed by the interaction of *mucins* (*glycoproteins* and *peptides* secreted by the *goblet cells* of the *epithelium*). It is an interlocutor space, which functions as a modern computer built of liquid crystals and provides us with immunological and energetic information.

    The dominant bacteria are chosen and privileged beings that live in the mucus itself, at the bottom of the intestinal crypt cells, and they take advantage of the benefits of living in a community (if they are noble and of good background). In reality, we take advantage of these bacteria even more: our intestinal cells use them for anything they need. It is an intelligent symbiosis that helps all to live well: one cannot be without the other.

- **SUBDOMINANT BACTERIA.** Another large group is the subdominant bacteria. They are somewhat repressed and used by the dominant bacteria. They don't have as much social influence or as many niches, but those they do have are stable residences that allow them to stay for a long time and to work with the dominant groups and the mucosa (again, if they are in the "good" group).

These two groups form the fixed, dominant community that defines whether the ecology of the host is "good" or "bad." Our yogurt—a loner and an optimist like Don Quixote—must arrive "in town" and be accepted into this community. If it doesn't manage to demonstrate its "nobility," allowing it to take its place in an intestinal crypt or position itself in the subdominant social groups, it will be classified as "bacteria in transit."

The majority of bacteria are bacteria in transit, in both variety and concentration, and they make up the most dynamic part of the microflora and intestinal ecology. These bacteria move progressively through the intestinal tract, mixing with the remains of food. They feed, interact, produce something good or bad for their "vehicle," and are finally expelled in the form of feces.

Most forms of yogurt and other fermented products contain "live bacteria" that will end up as bacteria in transit. They are like "tourists" that arrive in the colon to walk around, enjoy the local ambience, and later leave. However, in spite of just visiting, these bacteria influence the fixed bacterial society and the health of the intestine, in general. This "tourism" is beneficial for the colon, but in the short term. Bacteria in transit bring combustible and energetic properties and help to finish digestive processes. That is why it is recommended take probiotic products each day.

As you can imagine, if the permanent population of your intestine consists of "bad" bacteria instead of "good" bacteria, and instead of helping you attack you continually, lower your defenses, and inject toxins into you, causing inflammation, then the bacteria in transit can do little to improve matters. That is why I say, if you have dysbiosis it *must* be treated adequately; a pot of yogurt a day is not going to cut it! Only after treatment can you successfully maintain ecological equilibrium in your gut by eating functional foods.

The distribution of microorganisms in the different regions and zones of the colon varies in concentration and composition. The largest quantity of bacteria resides in the *cecum*, where transit is slower.

I want to say again: it is normal to have bacteria inside the gut. It may not be agreeable or sound refined, but it is essential. We are designed in such a way that the large intestine has the correct conditions to ensure prolific colonization of bacteria:

a more dehydrated environment that reduces flushing of microflora; a low rate of muscular movements of the intestine (peristalsis), a pH close to normal, and a great production of mucus facilitating the adhesion and nutrition of the bacteria. If the colon is sterile, the body easily develops serious allergies, reduced immune defenses, and the appearance of food intolerances.

If we cannot live without this diverse and enormous quantity of little creatures, it is better to work with them and understand this world in our innards. Over the course of our lives, bacteria regularly enter through the mouth and colonize our intestines. This is just a fact of life. So it is in our interests to control the quality of these "tenants" in our gut and to protect ourselves from any harm they may cause.

## Why Is "Good" Bacteria Essential to Our Well-Being?

What do the "good" bacteria in our gut do for us? Why do we need them? Here are some of the ways the biomass that inhabits our innards benefits us:

1. *Anaerobic bacteria* in the colon (meaning they can survive without oxygen) are responsible for metabolizing the carbohydrates and proteins we eat and, through fermentation, converting them into short-chain fatty acids (such as butyric acid). These short-chain fatty acids constitute the principal source of energy for *coloncytes* (colonic epithelial cells) and nourish the intestinal epithelium. Thanks to these bacteria, our digestive cells have food, can regenerate themselves, and can control their growth.

2. Bacterial by-products, including *acetic acid* and *propanoic acid,* play an important role in the liver's ability to regulate the metabolism of *glucose* (blood sugar) in the body by reducing *postprandial glucose* levels (after eating) and improving *the insulin response* (the vital hormone secreted by the pancreas and responsible for glucose transport, distribution, and cell nutrition throughout the body). Who would have thought that the quality of our intestinal contents would directly influence the metabolism of glucose? This is important in people with diabetes, who are overweight or obese, or who have various metabolic and hormonal disorders. The bacterial intestinal balance helps control the levels of glucose, insulin, and fats.

3. The fermentation of carbohydrates by bacteria helps us to better absorb important minerals and micronutrients such as calcium, magnesium, iron, vitamin D and so on. People who suffer from *anemia* (iron deficiency), *osteoporosis* (reduced bone density due to lack of calcium), memory loss, and disorders of

the nervous system, and who are always being advised to take iron, calcium, or magnesium supplements, can boost these vital resources in the body by improving bacterial transit in the colon, including in the cecum, and by taking care of their internal ecology.

4. Intestinal flora can synthesize biotin (vitamin B7), folic acid, and other B vitamins, as well as vitamins K and E. These are essential and important nutrients.

5. Intestinal flora transform bile acids and cholesterol into a great quantity of metabolites. The conversion of cholesterol into *coprostanol* by bacteria helps reduce total serum cholesterol. Some 80 percent of people with high cholesterol report that they have chronic or temporary constipation, gas, heavy digestion, or other digestive problem. Inevitably, this leads to dysbiosis. I have hundreds of clinical cases showing greater cholesterol control by simply regulating intestinal microflora and accelerating bilious and fecal transit.

6. Microflora in the digestive tract play an important role in the proliferation and differentiation of the intestinal epithelium. The bacteria that live in close proximity to the cells of our intestine help control of the growth and reproduction of the epithelium. They help control genetic expressions in the intestines, ensuring that they are functioning normally and without anomalies or mutations. Intestinal cells are exposed to *proteolytic bacteria* (putrefactive microbes such as clostridia that are a normal part of gut flora and secrete toxins such as ammonia), they can proliferate in an uncontroled manner, causing the formation of polyps (in some cases precancerous lesions) in the colon walls, which if not excised in time may lead to colon cancer.

7. Balanced intestinal microflora are essential for the development and maturation of a normal immune system, both *systemically* (the general defense of the body against external infections), and *locally* (through the intestinal mucosa). Distributed throughout the digestive tract are various types of *immunocompetent cells* (immune cells such as T cells that function normally following exposure to an antigen) and *lymphoid follicles* associated with the digestive system, similar to the tonsils. The good bacteria train the immune system to defend itself; they help it form and maintain immunological memory, competing with pathological and harmful bacteria for food and space; and they also nourish our mucosa. The balance of this system can be upset if the dominant and predominant resident bacteria turn against us. This often happens after a course of antibiotics or other

medications or as a result of chronic levels of stress or eating an unhealthy diet, and shows up as frequent infections, digestive problems, and general health disorders.

## How Can I Know Whether My Gut Contains Good Or Bad Bacteria?

How do you know if your good bacteria are surviving? Well, your gut talks to you through reports and symptoms. The symptoms of dangerous disorders come in many forms: bloating, gas, dark and foul-smelling feces, constipation, irritable colon, diverticulitis, polyps, Crohn's disease, colon cancer, and so on.

Primary or secondary immunodeficiency, malnutrition and, in general, chronic or acute debilitating illnesses can cause a breakdown in the equilibrium of the intestinal ecosystem. If you have any of the afflictions mentioned in this list, you will have to work diligently to ensure that the epithelial lining of your digestive tract is replaced regularly with friendly bacteria. If you are well and healthy, with regular bowel habits, you can maintain this state perfectly with diet, just as the adverts tell you. But if you are stressed, suffering from a cold, or need to take anti-inflammatories or antibiotics, even for a short period of time, I would advise you to do all you can to recover intestinal balance afterward.

One very common reason that the wrong bugs get a foothold in the "inner garden" is slow-down in the digestive system. On average, it takes food and nutrients (eventually becoming residues) 36 hours to travel through the digestive system, from mouth to anus. When the transit of food is slower or delayed (and in many cases, half blocked) this provides the opening for various unfriendly microorganisms to multiply and make themselves at home in the large intestine and influence its physiology.

As in human life, the more brutish, aggressive and ruder bacteria are, the quicker they become stronger, gaining territory and influence. Bacteria can reproduce so rapidly that they soon start to influence the metabolic activity of the whole system. Instead of this having a positive effect by activating our immune defenses and stimulating the repair of our digestive systems, all the "gifts" can become negative in the form of toxins, inflammation, fermentation, and so on.

Which kind of bacteria is winning in your gut? In the absence of serious systemic illness and antibiotic treatment, gut flora are normally stable. Epithelial cells in the mucosa with bacteria stuck to them are rapidly lost and the appearance of new epithelial cells that can be colonized prompts competition among different populations of bacteria to adhere to them. In such a situation, subdominant bacteria groups can be promoted to the position of noble, dominant bacteria, while bacteria in transit occupy empty niches and settle in for a long period. We have to be attentive, therefore;

always insisting on the use of functional products and supplements filled with "good" bacteria in order for them to dominate in the universe of the colon.

Antibiotics and other antibacterial agents, as well as chemotherapy and radiotherapy, may provoke significant disturbances in gut flora. The effect of antibiotics on the microflora depends not only on the scope of their action and pharmacology but also on the dose and its frequency and on the duration of the treatment. The type of host is also important: age, physiological and pathology of the flora, and an individual's reaction to changes in the body.

Alteration to the gut's anaerobic flora brought on by most antibiotics leads to an overpopulation and overgrowth of aggressive bacteria.. These resistant, aggressive, "bad" bacteria can then reach a critical population threshold, at which point they become virulent, causing diarrhea.

After a treatment of antibiotics or chemotherapy, the intestines can enter into a period of slow but stable recovery of their flora, or, depending on the physiological and pathological state of the person, there may be a chronic altering and unbalancing of the intestinal flora, marking the beginning of pathological and toxic processes in the intestinal tract. So as not to tempt fate, take probiotics and prebiotics during the chemical/pharmacological treatment, and for a period of two months after that, in addition to reinforcing your diet with functional foods.

Note: If prolonged courses of antibiotics or chemotherapy are necessary, it is a good idea to consume probiotics but they may not be very effective because they will be destroyed along with the pathogens during treatment. They may not die immediately, however, and in the meantime can do some good (such as, for example, balance the pH and nourish the intestinal cells). Think of them as kamikaze pilots who go into battle on short but effective missions. In times of war, when you have to kill almost everything to eliminate the bad, you have to take the risk.

To make everything clear, we will go over the terms again.

## Probiotics

You may be wondering how we learned so much about the positive effects of bacteria on the body. The history is quite interesting.

Starting with the early observations of Nobel Prize–winning scientist Ilia Metchnikov, the beneficial effects of lactobacillus and acidobacillus in human health have been of interest to scientists for more than a century. Metchnikov was the first to clearly establish that gut bacteria are not necessarily prejudicial to human beings; on the contrary, they play an important role in our well-being. In fact, Metchnikov was the first to advocate the consumption of live microorganisms and to realize that the role of lactic bacteria is to prevent putrefaction. In his opinion, it was this effect that was an indirect cause of the prolonged life expectancy observed in Caucasian populations that consumed large quantities of fermented milk products. Since then, considerable research has been carried out into what have come to be called probiotics.

The term "probiotic" refers to products that contain live microorganisms that survive the passage through the gastrointestinal tract and have a beneficial effect on the host (Fuller, 1991). Probiotic foods exert a positive influence on the health far beyond the energy and nutrients they contain. In particular, scientists cite various beneficial effects to be found in probiotic supplements, which contain strong living strains of "good" bacteria. It is worth pointing out that probiotics:

- reduce diarrhea of various etiologies
- reduce lactose intolerance
- improve the intestinal ecosystem
- maintain bacterial balance
- moderate immune system response
- improve antibacterial response
- protect against cancer

Probiotics administered to kids and adults cause changes to gut flora and its metabolic activity. Even though the changes they produce are small, when they are applied to pathological situations, they are often sufficient to beneficially alter the course of the illness. Probiotics are associated with an increase in the quantity of bifidobacteria and lactobacillus bacteria in the feces, lowering of fecal pH, and reduction in the bacterial enzyme activities that are associated with the development of cancer of the colon (Bezkorovainy, 2001, and Capurso, 2005).

## Prebiotics

Prebiotics are ingredients in food that are not digestible (principally fructo and glacto-oligosaccarides) and that selectively promote the growth and activity of a limited number of "good" species of bacteria. Prebiotics represent a preferred food for our good bacteria, an easy resource and a rich source of fuel. They are an essential nutrient to keep our friends alive and essential for good digestive health.

Food is key. It is obvious that you cannot maintain a balanced gut ecology with antibiotics, but neither can you do so if you overeat protein and refined fast carbs in processed food. You should nourish your good bacteria of gut microflora with prebiotics. When your friendly bacteria starve, they die. They are not carnivorous; they are vegetarian.

Prebiotics are indigestible carbohydrates consisting of dietary fiber that, after their transit through the small intestine, arrive in the colon practically without any modification. The best known prebiotic is *inulin*, a fiber that is found in great quantities in most legumes (pulses); in roots and tubers; in many vegetables, such as garlic, onion, artichoke, and cabbage; and in some cereals, nuts, and fruits, particularly prunes.

Inulin stimulates the growth of beneficial intestinal microflora because it passes through the stomach and the duodenum and reaches the large intestine largely undigested and unchanged. Here it is available to be metabolized by friendly intestinal microorganisms, such as bifidobacteria and lactobacillus, and so on.

# 11

# Gastroesophageal Reflux Disease (GERD)

Anyone with recurrent acid reflux undoubtedly suffers. It is a malady that appears after eating or drinking. Heartburn (*pyrosis*) is a burning sensation that rises in the chest behind the sternum. It can accompany either hunger or stress, with acidity entering the esophagus with any movement of the body. The condition is very disagreeable and persistent, and a great source of irritation. We have all experienced it at least once, and know how bad it feels. Common language captures the feeling well. When we say that a remark is "acidic," we mean that it is bitter, cutting, vitriolic, or caustic. GERD can feel that way. It is disturbing, and it is no wonder that we want to stop it using whatever method is at hand, usually over-the-counter medications.

GERD involves an increase in pressure over the esophageal sphincter, weakening its muscles preventing it from closing properly. The most common and obvious reasons for this are:

- Fast food, large meals, and overeating irritating and acid-causing foods
- Smoking
- Infection by Heliobacter pylori bacteria
- Excess consumption of alcohol and fizzy drinks
- Excess weight and obesity
- Pregnancy
- Chronic constipation, gas, and flatulence.
- Frequent use of anti-inflammatory and analgesic medications
- Disorders in eating behavior: bulimia, compulsive eating, binge eating
- Stress
- Food intolerances

Many people suffer from acid reflux disease without any obvious reason, though. So their medical histories have to be analyzed and previous occurences of the condition noted to identify the moment when the condition was triggered. In addition, a large number of patients have symptoms that are extra-esophageal (outside the normal areas of the digestive system), and as a result they do not get properly diagnosed.

Frequently, such people see their doctor complaing of problems with their lungs and respiratory system, including frequent respiratory infections, chronic coughs, asthma attacks resistant to the usual treatments, laryngitis, dysphonia, snoring, or erosions of the pharynx. It is not uncommon to confuse acid reflux with a heart attack. Also frequent in patients with chronic GERD are tooth decay and *halitosis* (bad breath).

GERD is a serious condition, one to which we should give careful consideration and try to treat. It leads to serious complications in the long term (as we shall see shortly) and is frequently not diagnosed early enough to prevent further problems. For this reason, GERD is considered to be the digestive illness that is the most frequent cause of morbidity in the population. Whoever would have thought that people could die of chronic acid reflux that hasn't been properly treated?

Remember that the esophageal sphincter is a muscular band similar to a fist that is positioned at the entrance to the stomach and is permanently on guard. It is very strong and very intelligent; it only opens to allow the food bolus to go down with a short muscular movement that is punctual and coordinated. If you put yourself in an upside down position, resting your weight on your head and your legs pointed toward the ceiling (a headstand), and then try to swallow some food or drink, or your own saliva, the esophagus and its sphincter will do this work as normal, generating a muscular wave toward the stomach, without producing regurgitation; in other words, without the contents of the esophagus returning. But obviously if your "fist" doesn't close well, you will "drown" in the acidic taste of the stomach juices that exit through your nostrils.

The condition develops little by little, frequently at a young age. Acid reflux and heartburn appear sporadically and typically go away without taking antacids or special foods; we normally blame this reflux on too much food and drink or intense stress. The mucosa of the esophagus knows very well how to recover after these transitory burns: it generates new cells, and the discomfort disappears. If any of the risk factors listed earlier persist, the digestive system puts up with them for a long time, compensating for the problems. Eventually, though, if subject to these same behaviors repeatedly, the esophageal sphincter loses strength and the ability to coordinate its movements: the sensation of occasional reflux and heartburn will become permanent, accompanying almost every meal. Over years and without any treatment, a light reflux can be transformed into GERD.

It is true that when someone has been diagnosed with GERD, it is very difficult to treat. You have to combine the appropriate medicine and nutrition in an intelligent way, along with supplements and exercise, and eliminate the main risk factors.

The incidence of GERD is rising worldwide. In the United States, GERD-related symptoms affect 15–29 percent of the adult population due to increasing rates of excess weight and obesity. In the United Kingdom, the rate is 21–29 percent. Across all developed countries, the figure is over 15 percent. Figures suggest that incidence of GERD is rising by 4 percent a year. Studies indicate that in the developed world, 15–22 percent of primary care visits are related to stomach problems, many of them GERD.

Around 20 percent of people with GERD develop serious complications, such as Barrett's esophagus (a precancerous change in the cells of the esophagus); adenocarcinoma (cancer) of the esophagus; stenosis (a lack of elasticity in the esophagus that brings with it a reduction in its diameter, impeding adequate swallowing); and acute or chronic digestive hemorrhage and ulceration. The incidence of these conditions appears to be increasing.

You cannot simply ignore GERD and do nothing about it, not only because of the consequences but also because of its effect on the quality of life. It can be treated using cyclical medical treatments, which can achieve a prolonged remission, without acute outbreaks and without the need to take medications for the rest of your life. Surgical intervention can sometimes be a radical and efficient solution. Gastrointestinal surgeons use a special plastic to remodel the sphincter area. It is essential to make changes to lifestyle and diet, avoiding irritating the mucosa and diminishing the pressure on the "new" sphincter.

### Why Do I Have Acid Reflux?

So that you can find the answer or at least a clue, I will give you some more information to add pieces to the puzzle.

On the one hand, we have factors that directly influence the sphincter muscles, such as bad habits and eating behavior, including:

- Not chewing properly
- Fast food
- Too much alcohol and sodas
- Aerophagia (literally, the "eating of air," meaning excessive swallowing of air, something that normally occurs when we talk as we eat, chew badly, and eat too quickly.
- Anxiety and compulsive attitudes toward food
- Bulimia
- Smoking

## Excess Weight, Obesity, Pregnancy, Constipation, and Flatulence

What could these apparently very different conditions have in common? A lot as it turns out. The abdominal and pelvic spaces are limited and shared by many organs. If an organ or a tissue grows and increases its size, the others will be affected. This "competition for space" leads to increased pressure inside the abdominal cavity, which, in turn, presses on the stomach (positioning it almost horizontally), flattening it and pushing it toward the diaphragm. As a result, the pressure on the sphincter of the esophagus naturally increases. This is the most common reason for gastroesophageal reflux disease.

During pregnancy, the growing uterus has priority in the abdominal space. Pressure from the enlarged organ and the "kicking" due to the movement of the baby, together with the influence of hormones, can cause very intense and unpleasant acid reflux. Although they are suffering, pregnant women put up with this and opt not to take medication in order to protect their babies. These assorted digestive sensations are frequently accompanied by constipation. Pregnancy is a trial by fire for a woman and her digestive system. After the birth it takes much effort and patience to recover her prepregnancy weight and correct digestive functions. But women do it, and they do it well.

Abdominal obesity, or overweight, is quite another subject. That round belly looks out on the world like a big face and completely covers the belt. In an obese person, fat occupies all the space around the intestines and stomach, covers the pancreas and the kidneys, infiltrates the liver with fat, and pushes on the bladder and prostate (or the uterus and ovaries). The interior world of the gut is entirely trapped and smothered in dense fat, and digestive and cardiovascular functions are altered by the buildup of pressure in the abdomen. In an obese body, the diaphragm is pushed up and inflated toward the thorax, and the gastroesophageal sphincter is placed under a great deal of pressure and can lose its strength.

In the case of chronic constipation, whether the person is aware of it or not, he is suffering from a buildup of compacted feces and gas in the colon. This organ is capable of adapting to the conditions by inflating, and can increase 10–15cm (4– 6 in) in diameter. Imagine that "hosepipe" housed in your guts reaching 2 meters and becoming that wide. . .

The colon may follow an extravagant route, spreading out its loops and folds in between its neighbors. The uncoordinated motility (regular muscle movement) provokes muscle spasms in the colon, and this in turn increases the sensation of bloating and flatulence. The tension inside the abdomen, and the pressure on the stomach and the sphincter, provoke acid reflux. It's worth repeating: a constipated intestine full of old residues can be the reason for gastroesophegeal reflux.

· · · · · · · ·

C. came to my clinic for a session of colonic hydrotherapy without having any obvious digestive troubles. In reality, she came at the insistence of her doctor, a colleague of mine.

She is a healthy woman, vegetarian and sporty. But at this time she had been off work for several months because she had lost her voice. She is a teacher, and her life is spent talking and teaching. Conventional treatments did not give her back her voice. She took omeprazole and some anti-inflammatories, and the doctors now saw the need to prescribe her corticosteroids.

She wasn't much interested in cleaning out her intestines but desperation and confidence in her doctor's recommendations guided her into my consulting room.

During the colonic cleansing, C. discharged from her colon an alarming quantity of retained residues, feces and gas, as well as an enormous quantity of worms. The poor woman was terrified to discover her insides were so unattractive.

Through a study of her intestines carried out afterward (a virtual colonoscopy) it was confirmed that C.'s large intestine was too long (megacolon), wide, and tortuous; it was not adequate for her constitution, and despite moving her bowels daily, she accumulated many residues and gas in her gut. Because she played sports and her abdominal muscles were strong, her belly didn't stick out, and she didn't feel particularly bloated. However, the pressure inside her abdomen was so high that C. developed advanced GERD (weakness of the sphincter) without having the classic symptoms of this condition. Stomach acid backed up and flowed into the upper part of the esophagus and managed to reach the larynx, affecting the vocal chords and burning them completely.

Medications took away her acid reflux and heartburn but not entirely; as the sphincter didn't close properly, and the pressure on it did not diminish, during the night stomach juices damaged the whole esophagus up to the vocal cords.

Curiously, in this case, the decompression and abdominal decongestion achieved through digestive cleaning had an effect on her lost voice. Correct maintenance of her digestive functions has now allowed C.'s diaphragm and stomach return to their anatomically correct positions, reducing the pressure on the gastroesophageal sphincter.

Her teaching voice has completely returned. Subsequently, with exercises and special postures, C. has taken control of her health and her life and she has not lost her voice again.

> Recovering the voice by removing excrement is a curious story. You never know how your digestive system will surprise you, so it is worth being attentive.

It is important to mention that acid reflux acts in a more aggressive form (provoking deep abrasive damage in the esophagus) if the level of stomach acid is very high.

## What Increases Stomach Acidity?

HELICOBACTER PYLORI INFECTION: This "superbug" beats out many others because of its survival and resistance. Helicobacter pylori infection is very frequent, very contagious and ultimately seems to be quite resistant to treatment.

This infection can be symptomatic or asymptomatic (without provoking noticeable problems); it is estimated that 70 percent of Helicobacter infections are asymptomatic.

In the absence of a treatment based on antibiotics, a Helicobacter pylori infection can apparently persist a lifetime. The human immune system is incapable of eradicating it. Fortunately, this infection is easy to diagnose. If you have gastric reflux that persists despite your diet and making necessary changes in your eating habits and have acute and frequent outbreaks of heartburn, it would be worth carrying out a diagnostic test. It is not a complicated test, and your GP can prescribe it. In general, infection by Helicobacter pylori affects the young, who are more exposed to the contagious conditions that lead to infection. It is so common that it can be enough to share food and drink, drink from the same bottle, or eat with the same spoon. Not to mention kissing!

Once diagnosed, Helicobacter pylori infection must be eradicated. I am a medical doctor who is devoted to naturopathy (ND) and generally seek holistic solutions for patients that have minimal side effects. On the subject of Helicobacter pylori, however, I am in agreement with the conventional medical position on treatment and opt for treating the infection with antibiotics. My first line of treatment is to eradicate this "superbug" and immediately tackle the side effects of the antibiotics by prescribing a treatment of probiotics, diet and a subsequent liver detoxication treatment to build the patient's resources.

FREQUENT USE OF ANALGESICS AND ANTI-INFLAMMATORIES: This is a complicated subject. Many chronic degenerative illnesses such as rheumatoid arthritis, osteoarthritis, fibromyalgia, lumbago, disorders of the sciatic nerve, various traumas, migraines, and many more bind the patient to long-term use of nonsteroidal anti-inflammatory drugs (NSAIDs) to deal with the unbearable pain of their condition. People who take

NSAIDs are aware of the side effects and often combine them with omeprazole, to suppress the production of stomach acid, which is the right thing to do.

We must remember that we have a pot of "killer acid" in the center of our bodies, in the stomach, that enables us to digest food and against which we have special protection (when it works). The cells that line the stomach are like soldiers that form dense lines and cover themselves with a strong alkaline mucus to defend themselves against the permanent attacks from hydrochloric acid. Every battle has its casualties. Each day, some of the soldiers die in the struggle and fall defeated into the abrasive soup. The little hole in the stomach lining that opens up when a cell dies has to be repaired immediately. Normally, that happens when the neighboring soldiers are alerted with a signal to "cover the breach with their bodies," producing even more protective mucus. The repair is almost immediate, and perfectly coordinated.

Molecules called *cytoprotective prostaglandins* (cell protectors) are responsible for issuing this alert. They are the agents that send out a warning and demand protection of the stomach lining. Curiously, as well as stomach prostaglandins, the body produces many other prostaglandins to manage different reactions and vital functions. The majority serve as messengers of pain, warning about inflammatory processes and "generating" the sensation of pain. NSAIDs block the production of prostaglandins in the body, thereby reducing pain. We feel relief because the messengers of pain are quiet (for a while). NSAIDs don't selectively block prostaglandins; they affect all of them equally.

What happens in the stomach to cause problems in this system? The repair cells don't get the message about the breaches in the ranks and the acid enters and burns these vulnerable spots. As a consequence, the mucosa of the stomach becomes inflamed (to the point where it can develop ulcers) and the sensation of heartburn appears: if the area damaged is near the sphincter, the inflammation can make its functioning worse.

What can be done? A classic solution is to accompany the main treatment with *antacids* (a group of medications that protect the stomach by controling the production of hydrochloric acid). This is absolutely necessary; even if it doesn't protect it totally, it undoubtedly suppresses the acid aggression locally. The future medications of choice will be selective anti-inflammatories that block the pain without affecting the cytoprotective prostaglandins of the stomach. These are already on the market. Another piece of advice: try to have pauses in the treatment, withdrawing the NSAIDs for a few days. The digestive cellular lining is believed to repair itself every four or five days. A possible way to help your digestive system to repair breakdowns is to give it some short pauses in the treatment. I repeat that I am talking about administering courses of NSAIDs in a cyclical form. Don't interrupt or withdraw any other type of medication (such as corticosteroids) without previously consulting your doctor.

**ACIDIC AND ACIDIFYING FOODS:** There are foods that, because of their molecular structure and the form in which they are metabolized, are transformed into acids and increase the acidity of the stomach and the body.

Normally the stomach controls the degree of acidity that is allowed to enter it by reducing its own acidity; however, when the stomach is inflamed (gastritis) or influenced by some kinds of medication, the acidification from food can unleash a more burning acid reflux.

We know *acidic* foods, such as citrus fruits and some other fruits, by their taste. However, we may be less familiar with foods that are *acidifying* (foods that don't seem to be acidic but are transformed inside the body into an acidic form). There are many of these: meat, milk, cereals, fats, fruit, sugar, cakes and pastries, chocolate, and so on.

Acidifying foods contain fatty acids, amino acids, trans fats (meaning fats hydrogenated with acid), and other food molecules that transform into acids during the digestive process. This doesn't mean to say that they are bad or that we have to suppress them; many of them are essential. What we have to do is to learn to alternate them with foods that are alkaline, such as vegetables and minerals.

We must learn that acid reflux is not "calmed" nor acidity reduced by drinking a glass of milk or orange juice or by eating a steak. To curb acidity, we are better off eating foods or taking supplements that have an alkaline content. Juice or puréed celery, carrots, new potatoes, fennel, parsley, artichokes, and other vegetables are ideal choices. Creamed vegetables can be very soothing.

If we are showing symptoms of acute acidity, we can begin simply with a pinch of baking soda (bicarbonate of soda) diluted in water. Try slowly eating an underripe, almost green banana, chewing it well, and drinking still mineral water at room temperature, in frequent small sips. Sometimes grain "milks" can help, such as those made from rice or oats.

Reflux and heartburn can disappear just by eliminating undesirable foods, or those which your body doesn't tolerate. I have seen many clinical cases like the one that follows:

· · · · · · · ·

In Europe, café au lait for breakfast is almost sacred and very traditional, even more so when you have breakfast away from home, in a coffee bar.

C. drank coffee like everyone else, although he always found coffee strong and aggressive, for which reason he diluted it with a lot of milk. Acid reflux and heartburn in the mornings accompanied him to work. He tried asking for little coffee and lots of milk, but he always ended up with heartburn. He tried organic, natural grain coffee, drinking it only at home; it still gave him the same kind of problem.

He gave up on coffee and opted for tea without milk, but every time he went back to café au lait he ended up with heartburn. He cannot tolerate fresh milk, not only because of its lactose content but also because of other components in milk (although he tolerates fermented milks better). By simply eliminating milk from his diet, he made peace with his acid reflux and forgot about his heartburn. Now he takes black coffee without having any heartburn or other problems. He has now changed his views: the aggressor that caused the acid reflux was milk not coffee.

# 12

# The Liver and Gallbladder

I confess that out of all the parts of the digestive system, the liver is my favorite. It fascinates me. The more I study it, the more it surprises me with its capabilities.

The liver may be compared to an intelligent "central processing unit" that filters, controls, and cleans a liter and a half of blood per minute and simultaneously processes around 500 vitally important biochemical metabolic reactions. Some of these processes involve the division and breakdown of chemical substances (*catabolism*); others, involve synthesis (*anabolism*), primarily of protein molecules. The liver is the body's processor of nutrients.

I have already mentioned that the liver acts as a purification plant for the blood. It plays a vital role in the detoxification and excretion of a great variety of endogenous and exogenous compounds. The liver is very fragile yet simultaneously a survivor: it regenerates rapidly and is grateful for care; it can regrow from just a tiny piece and function with only 10 percent of healthy tissue. Just 200 g (7 oz) of healthy or transplanted liver can save a human life, even if the entire organ weighs around 2 kg (4.5 lb) or, when it is full of blood, up to 3 kg (7 lb).

The liver deserves its own book, and it would be an honor to be able to write it one day. But for now we're only going to go over some of the terms and the basics of its functioning.

The regenerative properties of the liver made a famous appearance in Greek mythology, with the myth of Prometheus. Prometheus was, without doubt, the Titan who was most generous toward humanity, stealing fire from the King of the gods Zeus himself and distributing it as a gift among humans. For this, Zeus punished Prometheus by having him chained to a rock in the Caucasus, where an eagle picked at his liver every day. Every night, however, Prometheus's liver regrew at the same rate as the eagle devoured it during the day. His torture continued for a long time until he was finally freed by Heracles.

There are many references in both ancient and modern medical literature to the influence of the liver on our mood, emotions, and intellectual state. According to traditional Chinese medicine (TCM), for example, the liver holds "the soul"; it is associated with the fire element and it is considered more important than the heart, an organ full of energy and powers. The liver manages everything, including moderating mental activity. In TCM, it is thought that if *qi* (chi, our vital energy) is unable to flow along the liver meridian, it ends up concentrating in the organ and showing up as irritability, insomnia, depression, anguish, melancholy, and doubt. The phlegm gets stuck, and the mind clouds over. The gallbladder, for its part, governs decision making, courage, and cowardice. If a patient's gallbladder doesn't function well and accumulates bile, he will have a fearful attitude to life. For this reason, in TCM, cleansing (detoxifying) the liver is the treatment of choice for the maintenance of health.

Ancient Greek physician Hippocrates described four humors. One of them was the yellow bile of the liver. When bile doesn't flow, he said, it stagnates and is transformed into a thick black substance. The word melancholy means "black bile" and notably affects digestion and mood, altering the mental state of a person.

We use expressions such as "to be full of bile" "to raise one's bile," and "to spit bile"; and a comment can be full of "black bile." All of these phrases speak for themselves. If you are filled with rage and fury, if you have negative feelings and everything irritates you, you may be right, but don't forget your liver. Help it and encourage it a little, so that your bile flows.

When you clean out your liver you clean out your mind, as innumerable treatises of traditional natural medical wisdom from around the world affirm. Cleaning out the liver has a place in traditional medicine and is considered a very important therapeutic step. Following the development of modern medicine, we have lost the ancient tradition of draining and cleansing the liver to help the bile flow; recently, though, I have noticed increasing interest from doctors on this subject.

Unfortunately, when a patient is permanently sad, lacks enthusiasm, and is in an emotional trough (that is to say melancholic), a doctor usually prescribe antidepressants or tranquilizers and this, in its turn, increases the saturation and congestion of the liver.

As well as medications (if they are considered necessary) for the treatment of mood disorders, integrative medicine recommends the adoption of a light detoxifying diet, infusions of medicinal plants suitable for the liver, and cleansing the liver.

The liver is the largest organ inside the human body. It is situated in the upper righthand side of the abdomen, under the diaphragm. It receives a large part of the blood (85 percent) through the hepatic portal vein, the vein that drains almost all the blood from the intestine. This ensures that all the food absorbed goes directly to the liver, where it can be stored for use when needed, and that all the toxins absorbed can be filtered and deactivated.

The cells of the liver, the *hepatocytes,* produce between 500 ml (just under a pint) and 1500 ml (2.5 pints) of bile each day. *Bile* is a dense yellow liquid that circulates from the bile ducts (vessels) to the common bile duct. Later it is stored in the gallbladder.

The gallbladder serves as a reservoir for the bile secreted by the liver. Bile is concentrated tenfold by absorbing water, which is why it has a thick consistency and a dark color. The bile retained in the gallbladder can form a mud and condense the sands and crystals composed of bile salts. Over time, this mud can be converted into mineral *calculi* (stones).

When we eat, foods taken into the digestive system, especially fats, cause the gallbladder to contract, thanks to its muscular layer, eliminating the bile concentrated in the duodenum. Bile acids act as a detergent that emulsifies all the fats in the diet and facilitates their digestion and absorption. Without bile, we could not digest fatty meals, which leads to a sensation of having a slow and heavy digestion, bloating, and problems of intestinal transit at both ends of the digestive tract.

Another important component of bile is *cholesterol,* which is produced in the liver. The body requires healthy quantities of cholesterol, as it is used for various metabolic and regenerative functions. The remains of the cholesterol and bile acids that have not been used are eliminated with the feces. Curiously, a portion of these is reabsorbed in the intestine and recycled by the liver.

Occasionally, the amount of cholesterol produced by the liver and afterward reabsorbed and recycled can cause serum cholesterol levels to rise (sometimes with no correlation to diet or the consumption of fats). In such a case, a prescription related solely to dietary recommendations is not going to produce positive results: what is needed is to accelerate the elimination of natural cholesterol produced internally by the liver and to moderate its production.

If bile is not adequately expelled, due to a dysfunction of the muscles of the gallbladder (a "lazy gallbladder") or for other reasons, sedimentation, accumulation, and congestion of the liver with bile becomes apparent. This provokes a sensation of feeling full after eating; heaviness, as if "blocked up" inside; bloating and frequent constipation; and stools that alternate between greasy and foul smelling liquid diarrhea and hard feces that look like "goat droppings."

### What Causes Bile Retention and Gallbladder Problems?

The most recognized causes of bile retention and gallbladder problems are:

- Hepatitis
- Liver insufficiency
- Irregular meals, fast food, and a diet lacking nutrients, fiber, and essential vegetable fats
- Chronic stress

- Prolonged use of paracetamol, contraceptives, hormonal medications, and other drugs
- Excess alcohol and coffee

When we talk of a "fatty liver," we mean that the cells of the liver are saturated with fat (like liver paté) and that the *intrahepatic bile ducts* found inside the liver are full of dense bile with a high concentration of cholesterol (internal and external).

Fat accumulates in the liver because a person eats badly, is overweight or obese, has diabetes, or is on prolonged hormonal treatment; it also happens because of the recycling and assimilation of the body's own cholesterol and because of problems in the gallbladder. A liver full of fat cannot continue to adequately perform its many vital functions in the body, leading to problems in assimilating carbohydrates and fats and a worsening ability to carry out its detoxification function.

## Cleansing and Draining the Liver

During a liver cleanse, the liver is gently encouraged to improve its excretory function in order to eliminate old bile trapped inside the bile ducts and to achieve a complete and regular evacuation of the gallbladder. It is a delicate process involving the use of medicinal plants, supplements, mineral salts, oils, and certain foods.

Liver cleansing achieves the following objectives:

- First, the complete drainage and elimination of accumulated toxins, cholesterol, and other fractions of fat.
- Second, proper bile flow and improved motility of the gallbladder through dietary measures.

## What happens during the process of detoxifying and cleansing the liver?

The first phase of treatment involves several days spent preparing the body, using dietary measures and natural remedies, in order to soften the toxic and fatty materials in the liver. This helps them acquire a more liquid consistency, so that they can be expelled afterward and so that the bile ducts can dilate and relax.

At the end of this preparation phase, the gallbladder and liver ducts are encouraged to make strong and rapid muscular contractions to expel their contents by observing a day of fasting accompanied by the taking of certain oils and mineral salts. This daylong purging is profound and important, and it is not easy. It involves spending literally several hours in the toilet evacuating frequent jets of greenish, warm, foul-smelling liquid.

This amount of digestive activatation can be tiring. It can irritate the anus and lead to a sensation of weakness. This is to be expected, and for this reason it is recommended to carry out liver cleansing on a day free of appointments and to dedicate time almost exclusively to this.

The bile expelled during cleansing days is very dense and greasy, and has the consistency of clay or dark green "butter." After entering the intestines, it becomes knitted together (gets harder) and acquires various round forms similar to stones, which have to be evacuated and expelled within hours.

There is always a risk of recycling and reabsorbing these mobilized liver toxins; also, the "stones" are very heavy and sticky and often stay in the colon for a while; for this reason it is very important to carry out a good cleansing of the intestine (colonic hydrotherapy being the optimal measure) after the liver cleansing.

Sometimes patients observe multiple deposits of green bile in their toilets, and they even take photos of them! I have a gallery of such images on my computer: if only they could be prepared for an artistic exhibition, now that would be very original! Frequently, worms of all sizes are dragged out by the purge, along with fatty froth with the consistency of whipped cream and much sand. Some surprised patients, who are curious about their inner contents, fish out the little balls of bile and display them on a porcelain plate or in a sieve, comparing them to a coin or other object (all this I have documented, but anonymously, of course); other people tell me that they keep them in the fridge and want to show them to me in their natural form. I insist, however, that a photograph will do!

· · · · · · · · ·

J., 35 years old, worked in a fast food hamburger chain for more than 10 years. Obviously, burgers and fries formed his main diet during that time, and he didn't control the quantity of food and drinks he consumed over that decade. Luckily for him, he lost his job—he is seriously obese and has high cholesterol and problems with his digestive system.

Becoming unemployed was for him a blessing in disguise. He became fanatical about healthy eating and using natural complementary therapies. He has undertaken various cycles of bodily detoxification, including liver cleansing.

Astonished by all the positive changes he was experiencing, he decided to pay homage to the lost years among the hamburgers, soft drinks, and fries by gathering all of his liver "stones" (which, to be honest, is a great quantity) and has literally embedded them in the walls of the new house that he is finishing building in the north of Spain. A new body, a new life, a new house, and the "toxic" green memories, as he puts it. How can anyone not smile when they hear this?

Not only are bile and toxins moved, but also energy and emotions. Oriental philosophers have their reasons for pointing to the liver as the center of the emotions and the passions. Patients "uncover" their accumulated sadness and rage; they also feel very sensitive and very expressive during the day of the cleanse, and for several days afterward. One will start to cry for no apparent reason; another, at last, decides to let go of everything he is thinking. It is normal to feel sad and perceptive, more intuitive, and to begin to have more intense and vivid dreams. Without doubt, it is very useful and a great help to be able to share and talk about these changes with a professional psychotherapist.

One or two days after the liver cleanse, it is advisable to have a session of colonic hydrotherapy to ensure that any liver toxins that may have stayed in the colon are evacuated.

I repeat, according to theories of energy medicine, to drain the liver means to move, purge and discharge the emotions. After around two or three weeks, the first thing many patients report is an improvement in their digestion but also an intense emotional well-being, a more positive attitude, and a sensation of greater vitality; sincerely, they seem more happy.

I strongly advise you to carry out your first liver cleanse under professional supervision, and, after that, to learn to look after your digestive system and do annual cycles of detoxification (not more frequent). A badly-managed drainage can send hard mineralized particles through the narrow bile ducts and provoke colic. It can even manage to block the bile duct, creating an extreme situation that will send you to the emergency room of your local hospital. On the other hand, the toxic discharge of the liver can cause vomiting, strong headaches and fever, owing to rapid reabsorption in the intestine. Make sure you are protected from these complications by being properly guided.

In patients with a history of bile or nephritic (kidney) colics, or a history of these clinical symptoms, I consider it essential to carry out an abdominal ultrasound scan: this helps to dismiss the possibility of (or confirm) the presence of hard calcified stones that cannot possibly flow through the hepatic ducts when mobilized or change their form: these can generate great pain and lead to other complications.

It is also important to consider all other possibilities with a professional.

In recent years, liver and gallbladder cleanses have become fashionable, and I have hundreds of patients who come to see me after having done it badly, in an incorrect form, by relying only on popular books or information they have found on the internet. It is not a procedure to be carried out frequently. It is a question of well-being, of your health. Make sure you carry out the first steps with adequate advice, then you will learn how to do it and can do it by yourself. I remind you that naturopaths use many effective natural remedies for the liver. Look for the one that is right for you.

Remember that the adequate expulsion of bile depends on diet too. Medicinal plants and supplements to activate the liver should be taken just before or during the main meal. The most common natural remedies used for this process are: dandelion extract (root), green artichoke, Marian thistle, birch leaf, celery (the root is best), black radish, fumitory, turmeric, mint, rosemary, ginger, thyme, virgin olive oil, lemon juice, and magnesium sulfate.

A small but great testimony:

· · · · · · · ·

A., 34 years old. For many years (17!) I suffered the consequences of an illness that few people know about despite it being fairly common in society: bulimia. I tried different therapies and made little progress. My life seemed increasingly out of control.

Thanks to the therapy of colonic cleansing and liver cleansing, my body and my mind have been able to align. Now I can understand that my battle with food was not the real problem of my illness; I needed to reconnect with my body and my mind. Now I can enjoy and maintain my health and enjoy food.

## Liver Cleansing

### Days 1–5

#### AVOID

- Animal proteins: meat, sausages (and all processed meat products), poultry, fish, seafood, eggs
- Dairy products, including milk, cheese, butter (but you can eat fermented, or cultured, milk products, such as cottage cheese, quark, yogurt, kefir (better if they are made from goat's milk or sheep's milk)
- Fried and battered food, spicy food, sauces, mayonnaise
- Coffee (but decaffeinated is permitted), alcohol (all types), and tobacco
- Processed foods, including cakes and pastries, soft drinks, and chocolates
- Cold or frozen food and drinks

#### EAT AND DRINK

- Whole grains, fruit, vegetables, and pulses (legumes). All of these could be eaten boiled, raw, steamed, grilled, or cooked in the oven. Preferably

creamed or puréed, not fried!
- Cottage cheese, quark, yogurt/curd, kefir made from goat's milk
- Natural fruit and nuts, honey
- Water, tea, decaffeinated coffee, herb teas, natural juices, vegetable milks (made from oat, soy, rice, almond, hazelnut, etc.)

## REMEMBER

- Drink at least 2 liters of liquid a day.
- Eat small quantities of food (150–200 g) every 4 hours, or 5 meals per day.
- Eat slowly, chew well.

Snacks are essential mid-morning and in the late afternoon. They can consist of fruits, juices, fruit and nuts, yogurt, wholewheat biscuits, fresh cheese with sugarfree jam or honey, a mini-sandwich of wholewheat bread (with cottage cheese, mozzarella, tomato, avocado, and so on)

## NATURAL FOOD SUPPLEMENTS

(take for 5 days continuously)
- One liter of natural apple juice without sugar or preservatives (this can be bought in supermarkets or health food shops). Alternatively: 1 capsule (600g) malic acid a day, with breakfast.
- Celery and lemon juice (300ml). Dice 3 large celery stalks (preferably organic). Liquidize with the squeezed juice of one lemon, and add 200ml of mineral water. Alternatively: 2 capsules celery root extract a day, with breakfast.
- Epsom salts (powdered magnesium sulfate). Dilute 1 heaped tablespoon-ful in a glass of water (200ml). Drink in one go, after dinner. To disguise the bitter taste you can put a little honey or half a slice of lemon on your tongue before you take the Epsom salts.
- Powdered pysllium seed husks (*plantago ovata*) (one heaped tablespoon-ful) or a single-dose sachet. Dilute in 250ml of water (or apple juice). Drink immediately after the Epsom salts or a bit later at night, before going to bed. Keep the intake of this fiber supplement separate from your nighttime medication (one hour before or after).

## Day 6

**7 A.M.** On an empty stomach, take a heaped tablespoonful of Epsom salts diluted in a glass of water (200 ml) at room temperature. I recommend that you prepare this the night before. After you have taken this you can drink all the water you want.

**7:30 A.M.** Still on an empty stomach, mix 150ml of good-quality cold-pressed extra-virgin olive oil with the squeezed juice of two lemons (or the juice of one grapefruit). To mix it well put it in a jar with a lid and shake. Drink it straight away. To take away the taste of the oil in the mouth and throat, you can take sips of warm mint tea. Go back to bed immediately, lying on the right side and placing a warm blanket or pillow in the area of the liver. Sleep, or at least rest with your eyes closed, for 1–2 hours.

**9:30 A.M.** Still without eating, take a last tablespoonful of Epsom salts diluted in a glass of warm water (200ml).

**10:30 A.M.** You can now have breakfast (if you want). Continue with the vegetarian liver diet described above.

After dinner in the evening, take a tablespoon of the same fiber that you have been taking the previous nights: powdered psyllium seed husks (*plantago ovate*) diluted in 250mg of water or apple juice. It is important that you keep taking this fiber supplement every night for a week after the liver cleansing.

From day 7 on, you can eat a healthy, varied diet, as long as you care to eat high-quality foods and to respect your digestive system.

Within 2–3 days after the liver cleansing, it is highly recommended that you have a session of colonic hydrotherapy to eliminate any toxic and bile residues that remain in the walls of the intestine. It is also recommended that you take probiotics for a month after cleansing your liver and colon.

# 13

# Aging and Digestion

The changes that aging produces in our digestive system include:

- Weakening of the connective (supporting) tissues, with a reduction in elasticity
- Loss of muscle tone and resistance
- Reduction in the production of digestive enzymes and hormones
- Trouble with intestinal motility

Digestive illnesses related to aging and old age include:

- Hiatal hernia
- Intestinal diverticulosis
- Chronic atrophic gastritis, with a lowered production of hydrochloric acid
- Esophagitis

The whole body suffers degenerative changes with age, including:

- The skeletal system: osteoarthritis with wear of cartilage, disc herniation, sciatica-like pains
- The central nervous system: cognitive and memory disorders
- The immune system: immunological problems with a reduction of defenses.

Indeed, I am sure that some readers suffer from these problems without in any way thinking that they are people of advanced age.

Undoubtedly, factors such as traumas, genetic defects, nutrition and poor digestion, poor weight control, and related illnesses accelerate the degenerative processes, and with them the aging of the body. References to these illnesses and degenerative changes, especially in persons over 50 years old, are today appearing in the medical literature. However, 50 years old is not an advanced age! Agreed? It is not right to talk about infirmity and almost senility, when many people are living a very active life in their sixth decade, socially, physically, and intellectually. It is difficult to believe, but the body can have different ages on its exterior and in its interior.

Our society is getting older: the percentage of people aged 70 and over is rapidly growing. On the one hand, this indicates a better quality of life and social developments; on the other, the presence of large number of people who need specialized assistance—people who suffer from multiple health problems and who are on multiple medications.

It would be useful if our society looked after this increasingly long-lived population by increasingly understanding the importance of preventive care and making more use of alternative medications: these will enable older people to maintain their well-being and their quality of our life without resorting to drugs and visits to the doctor.

I would like you to turn your attention to early aging (premature aging), which is a reality and which is seen in many people who are relatively young.

Premature aging occurs when there is deep "internal wear" of the vital systems; prolonged cellular and hormonal dysfunction; when a person suffers from chronic nutritional deficiencies due to a bad diet, disturbed digestion, and limited absorption of essential nutrients; and lastly and very importantly, when the quantities of the toxic load due to internal toxemia or intestinal auto-intoxication and external chemicals, drugs, pollution go over permitted levels and overwhelm the body's ability to deactivate and eliminate them.

Premature aging corresponds to a collection of metabolic, hormonal, immunological, and degenerative changes. The functioning of these systems begins to slow down, and they switch off little by little.

Many people over 50 (and even younger) notice weaknesses and tissue wear and begin to be diagnosed with hiatal hernia, slipped discs, reflux, diverticula, osteoarthritis, adenoma, polyps, flaccidity, muscular hypotonia, and so on.

According to Iliá Mechnikov, winner of the Nobel Prize for Physiology and Medicine in 1908, the putrid fermentation in the intestine is the main reason for early aging and death. He introduced the use of fermented dairy products (yogurts) as a therapy to modify the defense of the immune system and to slow down the processes of intoxication of the body through its own residues. Mechnikov believed that he had found the solution to the problems of aging in the microbes of acidic milk. His theory and discoveries are still valid and coincide with the discoveries of modern medicine.

Constipation and the putrefaction of proteins are linked to the development of cancer and to premature systemic degenerative processes . It is absolutely certain that digestive equilibrium increases the defenses and regenerative functions of the body, and all this is related to youth.

## Cellular Aging

The biography of Dr. Alexis Carrel is difficult and complex to relate, due to the different facets of his personality that made him very controversial in politics and society. Winner of the Nobel Prize for Physiology and Medicine in 1912, he made important contributions to the development of the scientific bases of medicine and surgery, carrying out research in the field of transplants, tissue culture, and the theories of aging and death.

Carrel was interested in the phenomenon of old age and aging. He proposed the idea that all cells could continue growing, recovering, and rejuvenating themselves indefinitely. At the beginning of the 20th century, this notion achieved great popularity. Dr. Alexis Carrel was especially famous for an experiment he carried out on 17 January 1912. To confirm his theory, he placed a piece of embryonic chicken heart in a special flask and managed to keep the culture alive for more than 20 years! He did this by giving it regular supplies of complex nutrients and taking meticulous care of the cleaning and detoxification of the cells of the culture, changing the ambient liquid and controlling the parameters of the "environment." This gave a result much longer than the normal life expectancy of a chicken!

The experiment, which was directed by the Rockefeller Institute for Medical Research, received considerable attention, both from scientists and the general public. Dr. Carrel made a definitive contribution to the understanding of cellular regeneration and rejuvenation; in particular, the relationship between nutrition and detoxification, which was groundbreaking in his day. According to Carrel, the secret to the "immortality" of his experimental chicken heart culture lay in the strict maintenance of the parameters of the extracellular liquids. The solution containing the living culture had adequate proportions of highly nutritive compounds, optimal for cells and kept constant; the toxic products produced by the combustion and the functions of the cells of the culture were disposed of daily and substituted with a clean nutritive solution. The key to the success of the experiment lay simply in administering all the nutrients necessary and eliminating the residues in a regular and constant way. It is said that the chicken heart culture stopped functioning, sickened, and died when an assistant in the laboratory forgot to change the liquid (in which the piece of chicken lived almost eternally) for several days.

The message is clear, isn't it? If we look after our internal environment well (and in this I refer to the area of digestion) and we give it adequate nutrients (that is, we give it a balanced diet and encourage a productive digestive absorption), we have a high probability of living a very long active, lucid, healthy life.

In addition, as a result of all the studies of stem cells and biotechnological advances, it may be that in the near future we will be able to receive assistance and "be repaired" when we are confronted by problems or systemic failure. To reach this glorious moment of modern medicine, however, we have to begin to learn how to maintain and nourish our bodies, taking care especially of inner cleanliness.

### Aging is Reversible

The good news is that many degenerative processes in the human body are reversible! The design of a human being is very intelligent and almost perfect. It has an immense capacity to cure and regenerate itself and bring its programs up to date, if it is given adequate conditions.

From the earliest stages of infancy, each one of us confronts multiple toxins and certain types of cellular dysfunction, and the body immediately corrects them. With age, this ability to self-correct diminishes because the attacking forces overwhelm the body's defenses. Toxic accumulation in the body and subsequent discharge become imbalanced. It is as if truckloads of toxins (internal and external) are delivered to the cells and, in exchange, the process of elimination cleansing and discharge from the cells is carried away in vans.

If a cell is well nourished and hydrated, and the process of elimination and the de-activation of toxins and *free radicals* (by-products of metabolism) is adequately maintained, it can become almost immortal, or at least "young" and active for a long time.

A hiatal hernia or any other diagnosis that indicates the weakness and degeneration of tissues is a warning, a physical sign that you have to take up your own cause— get more active in the struggle, give more attention to your body from now on (not in the distant future), and that you have to take the necessary steps to delay and even reverse your premature wear and tear.

Life doesn't have to suddenly change. You do not have to make great sacrifices or abandon everything and escape to Tibet or move to the country. Small commitments to your health, such as half an hour a day of personal time and some kind of ritual related to your health, help a lot. You will see how your body thanks you for it.

## How To Start Your Anti-Aging Treatment

In integrative medicine, we treat the person not the illness. All aspects and functions of the human body are considered, and we do not only concentrate on a particular organ. For example, a patient with a chronic problem will receive the following holistic and integrated plan of treatment.

### Digestive Fine Tuning

First off, we clean and restore the functioning of the body's "most important pipe": the gut. Throughout this book, I have repeated the importance of digestive detoxification. To begin your journey toward rejuvenation, colonic hydrotherapy and liver cleansing will give you a burst of energy and will make you believe in your recovery and prolonged vitality.

## Strict Dietary Treatment

We undertake dietary treatment, which may include supervised fasts or special "half" fasts. As a professional, I find it interesting to apply various diets to improve the pH in the body, regenerate the digestive mucosa, and intensively clean and nourish the systems affected.

## Cleanse the Other Excretory Systems of the Body

In addition to the digestive system, we cleanse the body's other excretory systems, as these also eliminate toxins from the body. They include the urinary, lymphatic, respiratory, and integumentary (skin) systems of the body. This is accomplished using various natural remedies: inhalations, saunas, local cures, if needed, and a special diet.

## Supplement With Essential Nutrients and Functional Foods

We use natural products and remedies that do not have side effects to gently repair damaged functions in the body and improve the patient's well-being over time in noticeable ways. These treatments offer direct assistance from Nature, but require patience, trust, and dedication on the part of patients in order to stick with them. Taking these remedies and foods becomes a ritual, a daily habit, and over time a lifestyle. We do not place enough value on the healing potential of medicinal plants and natural remedies, in spite of the fact that modern medicine has its roots in their use.

For many people, a healthy life and youthful energy is synonymous with a life without stress—preferably away from the city, in the mountains or in a village with clean air—and consuming many organic products, being within reach of grandmother's natural remedies, and taking part in enjoyable physical activities. We may not be able to disconnect from the rhythm of urban work but we have at our fingertips many reminders of that pure and healthy life: medicinal herbs and plants that were gathered in Nature's garden. Medicinal plants enable us to maintain our health and well-being and reconnect us with Nature. More than half of people worldwide do not use pharmaceutical medicine, and not all of them live in misery or are unable to obtain Western medications; it is another way of living, simpler but also healthier.

Do you know that in Brazil around 90 million people have never used the medications and drugs that we habitually use in the West, and yet they stay healthy with only natural medications? They are not those people who live in the jungle, of course. Despite this, the average life expectancy in Brazil is 72 years. I'm not suggesting you go there. Nor am I asking you to abandon modern medicine and drugs. But I do ask you to open your mind and your beliefs to natural medicine. Dare to accept the ancient help of complementary medicine. As ever, though, I remind you that you must be assessed by a professional practitioner in order to safely use natural remedies.

## Restore the Equilibrium of the Intestinal Flora

Take the necessary probiotics and prebiotics to rebalance your gut ecology.

## Undertake a Personalized Program of Physical Activity

Every day, I hear myself repeating to my patients that they need to exercise. I know it is difficult to find time for a sport and that it is boring going to the gym and repeating the same routine. We find a thousand reasons not to exercise, to move our bodies, to avoid going to the gym or to an exercise class—even when we have paid for a gym membership or a series of classes every month!

The form of physical activity you choose needs to be fun, but you have to experiment in order to find one you like. What are you waiting for? Exercise: scientists say that we need to force ourselves to stick with the chosen activity for 21 days in a row, following a routine and doing it at the same time and same pace for the same duration in order to see results. If you do this faithfully, after three weeks, you will clearly see changes in your well-being and discover at last the pleasure and necessity of getting moving on a daily basis. Try it. Instead of being judgmental or long-suffering about it, try starting an exercise program with a positive attitude and strong determination to overcome your sedentary lifestyle. Physical activity is not optional; it is essential, if you want to maintain full fitness.

Regularly moving the body affects all of the muscular and other systems in the body. It stimulates blood flow through all the vessels, including the smallest ones and also improves circulation of fluids in the veno-lymphatic system and metabolic activity by burning excess calories and rapidly eliminating toxins.

You cannot drive your car at 120 km/h (75 mph) on the road in first or second gear. Agreed? If you accelerate like this, the engine will begin to protest and will have to work extra hard to keep the car moving. You have to put the car in at least fourth or fifth gear in order for your car to run as it is supposed to do and reach the right speed. Similarly, living at top speed in daily life, with its stress and tensions, without undertaking minimal physical preparation and training, is like advancing on the road of life and doing it badly—staying in first or second gear.

## Psychological Support

It is difficult to be all alone dealing with your problem or illness. You feel like you are the only one who is suffering. Nobody understands you. Everything irritates you. Sometimes you do not know how you go on, or who you should listen to. How do you manage your life when you're so tired and worn out? When we are sick or have ailments, we may feel that we are unique and the first to suffer, but that is not true. Our behavior and actions all conform to particular psychological profiles, and psychologists and psychotherapists are trained to diagnose these mental health conditions and to treat them. When we shut ourselves off in a world of suffering, unable to find a way out, this affects those closest to us. A trained therapist will work with you in a confidential setting to help you recover a positive and realistic outlook—both toward yourself as well as toward your problems. She will be able to guide you in recovering your emotional resources and mental clarity.

Think of your soul as an organ in the body—it too needs professional help to function optimally. It is of great help—I would say, essential—to receive a personal, family, or group psychological assessment when you are feeling bad. Unfortunately, in many parts of the world, seeking psychological support is devalued and many people find it difficult to share their worries. Psychological treatments may seem like a waste of time and money—unlike in the United States and certain European countries, where seeing a counselor or therapist is normal.

Do you remember when we talked about the different "brains" in your body, which manage your health and well-being, and how with a change in mental attitude everything changes? To overcome an emotional and psychological problem is not a question of will and planning your diary; it is something that you do not know how to do, and it is better to learn from a professional therapist. It helps all of your neuronal waves synchronize and come into harmony, so that you can continue the daily struggle with more clarity. Let somebody take care of you.

## Use a Combination of Western and Complementary Therapies to Treat Symptoms

I am not denying the need for medical prescriptions nor the use of drugs, if there is a real need for them. If there is pain, tension, or another problem, it is necessary to continue with the main treatment (which is designed to get rid of the symptoms of the problem) while working with a complementary therapist to improve your overall health. The use of complementary medicine alongside Western allopathic medicine to treat health issues is just around the corner.

· · · · · · · ·

F., 53 years old, is a healthy man without any history of illness. He is an aviation engineer. Three years ago, F. entered a midlife crisis; he also had personal problems and increased responsibilities at work. F. began to notice that his belly was pushing at the buttons of his waist and that he was suffering from insomnia as he lay awake doing calculations in his head. In a few months, F. discovered what it means to have acid reflux and heartburn, to not be able to digest food, and to be bloated. What most bothered him was the chronic fatigue that constantly dogged him (more faithfully than his partner). The tiredness would appear mid-morning and resulted in reduced productivity, which did not meet with the expectations of his boss.

He had a general checkup. The diagnosis: hiatal hernia, a malfunctioning esophageal sphincter and an irritable colon, and light depression. The treatment: four medications to be taken daily for an indeterminate period. Suddenly, F. found himself labeled an aging man (as well as a chronic neurotic) and rounded on his gastroenterologist with a thousand "whys?" and would not seem to accept reality nor his age.

Frustrated and depressed, F. looked for enlightenment in the health food shop in his neighborhood and there met a woman who insisted he buy a book about digestive cleansing. Enthusiastic, and without knowing anything about the subject of natural medications, F. tried many alternative treatments. Not all of them did him any good, but he has discovered a new world and improved his health a lot. He has learnt about healthy eating, yoga, and breathing. He has enthusiastically lost weight ... and his job.

When he came to my clinic, we organized a personalized program of treatments and health maintenance. Now this man seems to be full of energy and free of his ailments. He has new dreams—both professional and personal.

The typical treatment program that I have outlined above will demand a total of 2–3 months of discipline and effort to see noticeable and lasting changes. This is nothing in comparison with the years and decades that we can suffer from health problems. It is not a cure; instead, it is an opportunity for the body to reverse the pathological processes affecting it and to take charge of its defences and forces.

All of us—absolutely all of us—begin to notice the improvements and to acquire the taste for looking after ourselves. The body finds its center and regulates itself better, and it seems easier to control health problems.

• • • • • • • •

V., 50 years old, is a famous and beautiful actress. When I knew her, she had a life with much personal stress and was permanently weighed down by great emotional, social, and professional pressures. Despite her age and a serious medical history, she maintains her perfect appearance, but she was addicted to medications because of the chronic digestive problems that she had been suffering from for over 20 years.

Three years ago, we began V.'s personalized program of digestive and liver detoxification, as well as a program of functional nutrition. Since then, she repeats this annual program faithfully and is able to live without her medication, controling her digestion solely through natural remedies and diet. In her interviews, V. always says the secret of her energy and beauty is her inner cleanliness—and it is true, I assure you.

## Metabolic Age

In my work in the field of nutrition and dietary reeducation, I use modern medical equipment to assess and measure the bodies of patients. This gives me precise figures on the composition of their bodies, the quantity and quality of their tissues (muscles, fats, and liquids), and informs me of the risks and indices of their health. This program also calculates "the metabolic age"—the actual state of your body's functioning, nutrition, and cellular health in relation to the other readings taken. This is just a guideline. It gives a clear picture of the state of your current metabolic health at the time the readings are taken, and is subject to change.

I confess that I did not expect to make such a strong impact on people just by telling them their "metabolic age, but the truth is that your number in "metabolic years" can vary greatly from your birth certificate age.

In my consulting room, it is quite common to have women almost break down and cry when they discover that their metabolic age is 10–15 years older than their actual age, given how much they compete with each other, constantly diet, and weigh themselves over the course of each month. Men are equally surprised and overwhelmed to receive the same type of news. It scares them and gives them an incentive and a "kick" up the rear to do something about it and change things. I never imagined that this measuring instrument would be so useful!

There is a direct correlation between digestive upsets and a metabolic age higher than the chronological one; obesity can double the metabolic age and depression and the abuse of drugs more than double it.

The good news is that it is reversible! I have women who have lost 20 kg (44 lb) and gained 20 years of life in the bargain. Metabolic age readings drop noticeably after a program of detoxification treatments, after correcting constipation, and, in men, after losing abdominal fat. You also gain years when you exercise and maintain a positive outlook!

· · · · · · · ·

R., 47 years old, has complied with all the recommendations I have given her. She has lost some weight, changed her diet, begun to take physical exercise, and has started taking nutritional supplements. After two months, her nutritional and metabolic readings gave her a metabolic age of 38. I congratulated her and discharged her with the necessary maintenance guidelines. A few days ago she called my reception desk, and they told me that she insisted on having a medical certificate. I was surprised. After discovering the change to her metabolic health, she proudly told her partner and the people at work that she was only 38 years old and not 47. Nobody took her seriously, and worse than that, the poor woman was converted into the joke of the day. This is the reason why she wanted a medical certificate documenting her age of 38, recently acquired. Knowing patients who are so direct and naïve in their way of thinking puts a smile on our faces.

# 14

# Breathing and Digestion

In the middle of the torso, in the solar plexus, below the lungs and heart, the human body has a muscular separation that serves as the border between the chest and abdomen. This is the diaphragm. It looks like an unfolded parachute "supporting" the lungs and the heart. Below it are the liver (on the right) and the stomach (on the left).

The diaphragm is designed to be a very strong, resistant muscle that works tirelessly in synch with your breathing, descending with each inhalation and ascending as you exhale. If you are breathing correctly, on each inhalation (the intake of air) the diaphragm flattens and descends, leaving space for the lungs to inflate with the air; it presses gently on the liver and stomach below it and in this way massages all of the digestive and abdominal organs and stimulates them.

The free movement of the diaphragmatic dome creates a difference in pressure between two chambers: the chest (the thorax, or thoracic cavity) and the abdomen. This difference in pressure is necessary for us to have good circulation—not just the supply of blood but also the return through the veins and lymphatic system.

In the center of this dome (or the ceiling) there are orifices through which pass the esophagus (through a hole call the *hiatus*), large-diameter blood vessels, and nerve "cables." The circular-type muscles and connective tissue of the diaphragm around these "perforations" are lighter and delicate—these areas of greatest weakness where a hernia may form. With each inhalation the diaphragm descends, helping to propel the contents of the stomach on their journey through the esophagus and preventing them from returning and causing acid reflux (regurgitation).

For this reason, I consider it essential to learn to breathe and to do breathing exercises in order to have good digestive health. Respiration is a powerful tool. It can help prevent acid reflux, hiatal hernia, bloating, and intestinal spasms and control transit through the intestine.

Observe your breathing. How is it? Normally, breathing is something obvious, comfortable, simple, automatic, and involuntary; it doesn't need our mental control. Now I want to ask you for your full attention and to observe your respiratory rhythm.

What movements are there when you are peaceful and quiet? Do you notice the gentle, barely noticeable rising and falling of the chest—generally, in the upper part of the thorax, at the level of the arms or breasts? And how is the gut? The most likely answer is that it is "sleeping and relaxed" and that "it doesn't breathe or participate in the process." The abdominal area seems to be excluded from the act of respiration because it hardly moves at all, neither with the entrance nor the exit of air. It greatly satisfies us not to bother the belly; normally we always we give it a preferential space. When seated, we lean back slightly, supporting the back, so as to leave the stomach free, without pressing too much on it or squashing it.

How does your respiratory process change when you suddenly speed it up through physical activity, or when you are affected by stress, have a cold or fever, or you become passionate or excited? In these situations, respiratory movements become more frequent, superficial, and visible, because they involve a number of muscles in the process—the whole chest, arms, neck, and partly, the belly—but you will still note that the major part of respiration takes place essentially in the chest. Remember how ladies breathed in old films, elegantly attired in their low-cut dresses? This is a kind of breathing that we are going to call *pectoral*.

Now we're going to turn our attention to *abdominal or diaphragmatic breathing*. This involves the respiratory movements of the diaphragm and the abdominal wall. Here, the energy is centered in the area of the navel, which means that with this type of respiration, the chest doesn't visibly move as much with the rhythm of respiration and the intestines are more involved, as the abdomen inflates and deflates continually. To train yourself to automatically do belly breathing, as it is often called, is key to health, and not only to digestive health. Through it you can activate and oxygenate literally the whole of your body.

During inhalation, the belly should swell slowly, like a balloon, rising like a mountain; during exhalation, it should help eliminate all of the air, forming a hollow or a valley. In traditional Chinese medicine, and in particular the practice of qigong (chi kung), conscious abdominal respiration is the basis of cure and of energetic balance.

The benefits of diaphragmatic breathing are many. It is, above all, a magnificent way to relax the body and mind. It appears that greater circulation in the veins and the lymphatic vessels produces a continual massage of the abdominal organs and contributes to digestive health. Each abdominal inhalation generates a vacuum that "sucks" the intestines upward, along with the abdominal wall, and it relaxes them with each exhalation. This is the best way to stimulate intestinal motility and relax spasms. The difference in pressure that is generated at the peak of inhalation accelerates the filling and the irrigating of the organs with oxygenated blood; and during the descent, the exhalation, it promotes discharge through the veins and lymphatic vessels that, in turn, can be of great help in reducing hemorrhoids.

On the other hand, the vacuum generated during inhalation and the movement of the diaphragm center pushes the liquid contents of the stomach and the intestines toward the navel, helping in this way to improve the digestive enzyme processes and prevent reflux.

A study was carried out in an Australian IT and accountancy firm, in which the staff were asked to take a break for two minutes for every three hours of work. During these two minutes, employees had to practice exercises of abdominal breathing and relaxation. Two minutes without getting up from your chair! These exercises permitted employees to better oxygenate their whole bodies and stimulate their circulation and digestion. The result was an improvement in well-being, energy, mood, and intellectual productivity. In fact, I have personally seen advertisements in the Australian press that remind people of the necessity to restore their energy and to take pauses in order to breathe well.

You don't have to constantly pay attention to your breathing or try to control it or change it from one day to the next. I suggest, instead, that you adopt a ritual, your small personal space within the day, a moment in which you can "stop the world," disconnect, make yourself comfortable, and be peaceful for 10–15 minutes. I ask you to dedicate this time only to your breathing. If you want, you can consider it as a form of meditation or as a ritual/exercise of full consciousness; the power to be completely in the "here and now." Below is an example of how you can do it.

## Full Breathing

First, prepare yourself mentally. Think of this as a moment only for you, the benefits of which will be shared with everyone else. You deserve a moment of peace, tranquility, and well-being. If possible, especially when you are learning, choose a comfortable place.

Your posture should be relaxed, but keep your back straight.

If you can, adjust the lights, put on relaxing music, light a candle or incense, or simply imagine that you are in a beautiful place.

Unfasten your belt and any other item of clothing that feels tight.

Make sure there are no interruptions.

If in any moment during this exercise, you experience a sensation of being short of breath or dizzy, return to breathing normally.

Close your eyes.

Concentrate on your breathing.

Notice the air that you breathe in and the air that you breathe out.

For the first four or five breaths, don't make any changes. Just observe them.

Then inhale slowly through the nose and direct the air to the bottom part of the abdomen, around the area of the navel, perceiving and visualizing the lowering of the diaphragm.

The belly inflates and the diaphragm moves, allowing the thoracic cavity to expand, but the chest and the shoulders should not move.

Continue to inhale and feel how the breath reaches the middle and finally the upper part of the lungs, until the chest expands fully.

Hold the breath for a few seconds, without force or tension.

Now let it exit slowly through the mouth.

Let it first deflate the upper part of the lungs, then the middle, and finally the stomach, while you think, "I am feeling good. I am relaxed." You can help yourself by putting one hand on the area of your navel and the other on your chest.

On breathing in, the hand on your chest shouldn't move until the belly has filled with air.

On breathing out, the hands on the chest should go down first, followed by the one on the stomach.

Repeat the exercise 5–10 times.

Do this at least twice a day, in the morning when you get up and at night before you go to bed, until you manage to make it a natural, fluid, and relaxing rhythm.

Remember that this is how babies breathe—which means that we have all breathed like this once. Recover it!

When the air reaches your lungs, imagine that it is golden air or luminous, healing energy. Observe your breathing and think about this golden air.

Feel it.

Follow its path through you.

When it leaves your body, see how it takes with it all the tension.

Your body loosens up.

Imagine that you are a rag doll. Your body feels warm, light, or heavy. It feels relaxed.

When you feel that you can do this exercise in a fluid and easy manner, do it with your eyes open in whatever place you find yourself, except when you're driving.

# Final Comments

Dear reader,

This book has taken you on a first journey through your digestive world, with the aim of identifying some problems and disorders, clarifying terms, giving a better sense of orientation within the territory of your gut, and, most importantly, enabling you to appreciate the intelligence of your digestive system in all its aspects:

- Intelligence in its design and perfection.
- Intelligence in acting as a second brain, the enteric nervous system.
- Intuitive intelligence and gastrointestinal emotional intelligence, with its many facets.
- Digestive intelligence, which resists and protests against the "mistreatment" to which we sometimes subject it, shouting at us and obliging us to make changes
- Intelligence in its independence, its digestive autonomy, that doesn't adhere to social rules or care about human prejudices. It is authentic and is perhaps capable of expressing how you really feel in this moment. It is the most sincere part of you that escapes the control of the mental "police."
- Intelligence in the way it defends you against infection and provides you with the nutrients you need.
- Intelligence of inter-relationships. Your intestines know how to benefit from their billions of occupants and invaders, even if you don't know how.

Many other themes and problems related to our digestive systems could be discussed. I hope be able return to you soon with more information and practical advice. I hope, however, I have given you the pleasure of getting to know your innards, shown you a new world hidden in your body, awoken your interest it, and encouraged you to respect your digestive system, becoming aware of your diet, habits, and lifestyle—and perhaps convinced you to take the first steps toward becoming or remaining healthy.

This has been the first class. I hope to see you soon for the second lesson, so that you may learn to identify more with your symptoms and take the correct measures to deal with them. This does not seem like the right time to cover all the different templates of treatment available. Each of us is a unique world that needs to be treated in a personalized way.

If I have managed to motivate you to look for a practitioner of holistic medicine through reading this book, I will be delighted.

This book does not offer facts in order to challenge allopathic medicine, and it is not meant as a substitute for a consultation with a medical doctor specializing in working with the digestive system. My aim here is to assist such doctors in educating their patients about the care of their digestive system. To know your own aches and pains and understand the expressions and tricks of your body; to have a grasp of the necessary basics of diet and the care of the digestive system: all this contributes to good health and improving the quality of life of many people. At least allow me to keep this hope.

I will be delighted to receive suggestions, comments, and questions via *www.irinamatveikova.com*.

See you soon.
Irina

# Bibliography

**BOOKS**

Albers, Susan. *Eating Mindfully: How to End Mindless Eating and Enjoy a Balanced Relationship with Food.* Oakland, CA: New Harbinger Publications Inc, 2003.

Anderson, Rich. *Cleanse & Purify Thyself.* Medford, OR: Christobe Publishing, 2007.

Andreoli, Thomas, et al. *Andreoli and Carpenter's Cecil Essentials of Medicine.* Eighth edition. Philadelphia, PA: Saunders Elsevier, 2010.

Arem, Ridha. *The Thyroid Solution: A Revolutionary Mind-Body Program for Regaining Your Emotional and Physical Health. New York:* Ballantine Books, 2007.

Balch, Phyllis and James. *Prescription for Nutritional Healing.* New York: Penguin Putman Inc, 2000.

Beningaza de Hernández, Gloria. *Hidroterapia colónica,* Buenos Aires, Argentina: Ediciones La Casa de Silvana, 2004.

Bichen, Zhao. *Tratado de alquimia and medicina taoísta.* Madrid, Spain: Miraguano Ediciones, 1984.

Bittman, Mark. *Food Matters: A Guide to Conscious Eating.* New York: Simon & Schuster, 2009.

Borysenko, Joan. *Inner Peace for Busy Women.* Carlsbad, CA: Hay House Inc, 2003.

Bravo Díaz, Luis. *Farmacognosia.* Madrid, Spain: Elsevier España, 2003.

Fetrow, Charles W. and Ávila, Juan R. *Complementary & Alternative Medications.* Ambler, PA: Springhouse Publishing Co., 2001.

Gershon, Michael D. *The Second Brain.* New York: HarperCollins Publishers, 2003.

Gesner, Conrad. *Tesoro de los remedios secretos de Evónimo Filiatro.* San Lorenzo de El Escorial: Estudios Superiores de El Escorial, 1996.

Gray, Juliet. *Carbohydrates: Nutritional and Health Aspects.* Belgium: ILSI Europe, 2003.

Hernández Ramos, Felipe. *Que tus alimentos sean tu medicina.* Barcelona, Spain: RBA Libros, 2003.

Jensen, Bernard. *Dr. Jensen's Guide to Better Bowel Care. A Complete Program for Tissue Cleansing Through Bowel Management.* New York: Avery/Penguin Putnam Inc, 1999.

Johnson, I.T. and Southgate, D.A.T. *Dietary Fiber and Related Substances.* London, UK: Chapman and Hall, 1994.

Joshi, Nish. *Joshi's Holistic Detox.* London, UK: Hodder & Stoughton, 2006.

Junger, Alejandro MD. *Clean*. New York: HarperCollins, 2009.

Kabat-Zinn, Jon. *Coming to Our Senses: Healing Ourselves and the World Through Mindfulness, New York: Hyperion,* 2006.

Kaptchuk, Ted J. *The Web That Has No Weaver: Understanding Chinese Medicine*. Second edition. New York: McGraw-Hill, 2000.

Kligler, Benjamin and Lee, Roberta. *Integrative Medicine: Principles for Practice*. New York: McGraw-Hill, 2004.

Kumar, Nagi B. *Integrative Nutritional Therapies for Cancer: Facts and Comparisons*. New York: Springer, 2012.

Lagarde, Claude. *Votre santé se cache au coeur de vos cellules: découvrez la nutrition cellulaire active*. Saint-Julien-en-Genevois, Switzerland: Editions Jouvence, 2008.

Lawless, Julia. *The Complete Illustrated Guide To Aromatherapy*. London, UK: Element, 1997.

Lipski, Elizabeth. *Digestive Wellness: Strengthen the Immune System and Prevent Disease Through Healthy Digestion*. Fourth edition. New York: McGraw-Hill, 2011.

Medsker, Bekki and D. *Understanding the Need for Colon Hydrotherapy*, Quinsby: Medsker Publishing, 1997.

Moritz, Andreas. *Timeless Secrets of Health and Rejuvenation*. Fifth edition. Brevard, NC: Ener-Chi Wellness, 2009.

Ody, Penelope. *Complete Guide to Medicinal Herbs*. Second edition. *London, UK: Dorling Kindersley*, 2000.

Olsen, Cynthia. *ESSIAC: A Native Herbal Cancer Remedy*. Pagosa Springs, CO: Kali Press, 1998.

Pagano, John O. A. *Healing Psoriasis: The Natural Alternative*. Englewood Cliffs, NJ: The Pagano Organization, 2004.

Pengelly, Andrew. *The Constituents of Medicinal Plants*. Oxford, UK: CABI Publishing, 2004.

Pérez-Calvo Soler, Jorge. *Nutrición energética and salud*. Barcelona, Spain: Grijalbo, 2009.

Pipher, Mary. *Hunger Pains: The Modern Woman's Tragic Quest for Thinness*. New York: Ballantine Books, 1997.

Roth, Geneen. *Breaking Free from Emotional Eating. London, UK:* Plume, 2003

——.*Women Food and God: An Unexpected Path to Almost Everything. London:* Simon & Schuster, 2010

Satz, Mario. *Música para los instrumentos del cuerpo*. Madrid, Spain: Miraguano Ediciones, 2000.

Sears, Barry. *Toxic Fat*. Nashville, TN: Thomas Nelson, 2008.

Servan-Schreiber, David. *Anticancer: A New Way of Life*. Paris, France: Robert Laffont, 2007.

Schwartz, Mark S. *Biofeedback*: *A Practitioner's Guide*. Third edition. New York: Guilford, CT: 2006.

Steiner, Rudolf. *Nutrition: Food, Health, and Spiritual Development. Forest Row, UK:* Rudolph Steiner Press, 2009.

Thomson. *Physicians Desk Reference for Herbal Medications*. Fourth edition. Montvale, NJ: Thomson Healthcare, 2007.

Ullrich, Manfred A. *Chronische Krankheiten durch Colon-Hydro-Therapie erfolgreich behandeln. Baunach, Germany:* Spurbuch Verlag, 2011.

Vasey, Christopher. *The Naturopathic Way: How to Detox, Find Quality Nutrition, and Restore Your Acid-Alkaline Balance*. Rochester, MA: Healing Arts Press, 2009

Whang, Sang. *Reverse Aging*. Miami, FL: JSP Publishing, 2004.

Young, Robert and Redford Shelley. *The pH Miracle, Wellness Central*. New York: Warner Books, 2002.

## PERIODICALS

Bezkorovainy, Anatoly. "Probiotics: determinants of survival and growth in the gut." *American Journal of Clinical Nutrition*, vol. 73, February 2001, 399-405.

Capurso, G, Marignani, M and Delle Fare, G. "Probiotics and the incidence of colorectal cancer: when evidence is not evident." *Atti Abstracts*, 3º Probiotics & Prebiotics. New Foods, September 4/6, 2005.

Fuller, R. "Probiotics in human medicine: progress report." *GUT,* 1991, 32, 439-442.

# About the Author

Irina Matveikova, MD, is a Spanish board-certified family medicine physician. She specializes in Endocrinology and Clinical Nutrition and is a certified expert in Eating Disorder Behaviors.

After graduating from medical school, Dr. Matveikova undertook postgraduate professional studies (as well as studies in natural and holistic medications) in many different parts of the world, including France, the United States, Argentina, Spain, and the Czech Republic. She has extensive international experience of professional teaching in medical institutions and foundations, where she has given both conferences and classes.

As a result of her postgraduate experiences, Dr. Matveikova became a staunch believer in harmoniously combining natural and conventional medical approaches to health and is now at the forefront of this field. She is the author of numerous published articles about digestive health and functional nutrition. In addition, she recently (January 2013) published her new book in Spanish, *Salud Pura* (*Pure Health*), a practical natural health and detox manual and a followup to *Digestive Intelligence*. She is currently working on a new book project in Spanish titled *Digestive Intelligence for Kids,* which will be published in fall 2014. Irina Matveikova, MD, also has written a book of children's stories (fairy tales) about natural plants and foods and a dictionary of medicinal plants (in five languages) that, so far, are unpublished.

Dr. Matveikova's practice focuses on Integrative, Holistic, and Preventive medicine and places great emphasis on the self-education of patients. She has received wide recognition and acknowledgment as a reference and opinion leader in her field throughout Spain and Latin America, where she is regularly quoted in leading newspapers and magazines. She is frequently invited to be a guest on many prime time TV and broadcast programs in those countries.

Dr. Matveikova has been invited to head conferences in various public and professional institutions throughout Spain, and to participate in celebrity book signings at national book fairs.

She works from her own private medical clinic in the center of Madrid, as well as traveling extensively to many other parts of the country for external consultations.

# Index

FINDHORN PRESS

*Life-Changing Books*

For a complete catalogue,
please contact:

Findhorn Press Ltd
117-121 High Street,
Forres IV36 1AB,
Scotland, UK

*t* +44 (0)1309 690582
*f* +44 (0)131 777 2711
*e* info@findhornpress.com

or consult our catalogue online
(with secure order facility) on
www.findhornpress.com

For information on the Findhorn Foundation:
www.findhorn.org